DIABETES:
RECIPES FOR HEALTH

Executive Editor: Richard A. Weimer
Production Editor/Text Designer: Michael J. Rogers
Art Director: Don Sellers, AMI
Typesetting by: Carver Composition, Arlington, VA
Typefaces: Century Schoolbook (text) and Souvenir (display)
Printed by: R. R. Donnelley & Sons Company, Harrisonburg, VA

DIABETES:
RECIPES FOR HEALTH

Ann VonderHaar Christy, RD   **Judy Dvorak Germann, RN**

Robert J. Brady Company
A Prentice-Hall Publishing and Communications
Company
Bowie, Maryland 20715

Diabetes: Recipes for Health

Library of Congress Cataloging in Publication Data

Christy, Ann.
  Diabetes, recipes for health.

  Bibliography: p.
  Includes index.
    1. Diabetes—Diet therapy—Recipes.   I. Germann, Judy Dvorak.
II. Ehlen, K. J. (K. James)   III. Title.
RC662.C47   1982   616.4'620654   82-16438
ISBN 0-89303-211-5

Prentice-Hall International, Inc., London
Prentice-Hall Canada, Inc., Scarborough, Ontario
Prentice-Hall of Australia, Pty., Ltd., Sydney
Prentice-Hall of India Private Limited, New Delhi
Prentice-Hall of Japan, Inc., Tokyo
Prentice-Hall of Southeast Asia Pte. Ltd., Singapore
Whitehall Books, Limited, Petone, New Zealand
Editor Prentice-Hall Do Brasil LTDA., Rio de Janeiro

Printed in the United States of America

83 84 85 86 87 88 89 90 91 92   10 9 8 7 6 5 4 3 2 1

CONTENTS

FOREWORD

The purpose of this book is to provide you with guidelines for the successful day-to-day management of diabetes. Health and happiness as well as survival are possible for the diabetic and this book gives you the guidelines, as well as everyday, ethnic, and holiday recipes, that will help you attain a happy, healthful lifestyle. The cornerstone for diabetic care is a solid understanding of diabetes by the individual and those close to him or her. In this book such an understanding can be found for both the recently diagnosed diabetic as well as the established diabetic who is refreshing his or her information.

The material found in *Diabetes: Recipes for Health* comes from the experience of the Diabetic Teaching Program at Metropolitan Medical Center in Minneapolis, Minnesota over the last 15 years. An effort to teach about diabetes in a way that all can understand is reflected in this book. It has been widely recognized for its easy-to-understand approach and is being used in other hospitals and teaching centers throughout the United States. The hallmark of this effort is the precise, simple language and entertaining and highly informative diagrams.

Our understanding of diabetes is broadening rapidly. It is important to make an effort to stay as current as possible with this understanding. This book attempts to bring the reader up to date with recent advances in diabetic care and it reflects the efforts of the American Diabetes Association to maintain many widely available resources for the diabetic and those that help care for diabetics. *Diabetes: Recipes for Health* is meant for regular, repetitive use and it is hoped that it helps to permit happy, healthful survival for the diabetic.

K. James Ehlen, MD

I

HEALTHY LIVING

1
Putting The Pieces Together

WHAT IS DIABETES?

Diabetes mellitus is a chronic disease condition in which your body uses sugar improperly. Diabetes affects many parts of the body. It may lead to early aging of the blood vessels of the eyes, kidneys, heart, and lower legs.

No one is sure what causes diabetes. In the type of diabetes called Type I, doctors know that certain cells of the pancreas stop producing insulin. Insulin is a substance that helps our bodies use food. Recent studies show that a virus may damage these cells. Usually, this happens in people under 40 years of age.

The more common type of diabetes, called Type II, is often linked to a family trait or obesity. The cells making insulin slowly make less and less insulin. Another possibility is that the insulin made no longer works in the body as it should. Persons who seem most likely to get diabetes are those:

- with a family history of diabetes
- who are obese
- who are under stress (illness, pregnancy, surgery, infection, or emotional strain)

You are also more likely to get diabetes as you grow older.

To understand what occurs when a person has diabetes, let's first look at what happens to food eaten by persons who do not have diabetes.

Almost all of the food that we eat is changed into glucose by our bodies. Glucose, or sugar, is needed by the body for energy. You might consider sugar or glucose the body's fuel.

3

When we eat food, sugar enters our bloodstream. The normal level of blood sugar is 70–110 milligrams of sugar per 100 milliliters of blood (mg%). As this level goes up, the pancreas begins to send insulin into the bloodstream. Insulin allows our body to use our blood sugar for energy.

The following diagrams show you how insulin lets the body use sugar.

1. This is an enlarged drawing of a blood vessel. Close to the blood vessel are cells. Our bodies are made up of billions of cells; each cell works constantly to turn sugar into energy. Cells have walls which control what will enter and leave the cell.

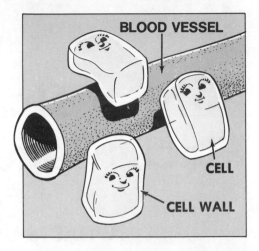

2. When we eat, food is changed into sugar and enters the bloodstream.

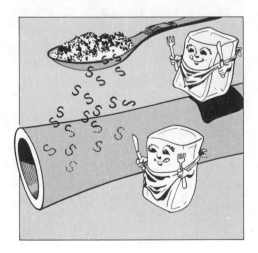

3. When the blood sugar level begins to go up, a message is sent to the pancreas. This message tells the pancreas to send insulin into the bloodstream.

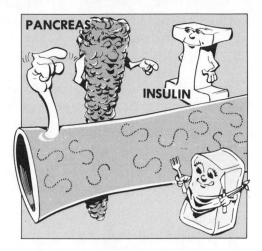

4. Insulin opens the cell wall, just like a key opens a door. Sugar from the bloodstream moves into the cell.

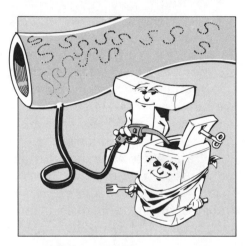

5. The cell can then produce energy for walking, talking, thinking, work, and fun . . . everything!

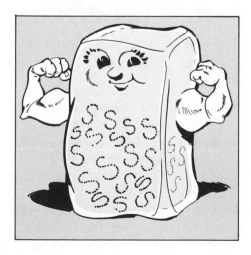

In the diabetic person, the cell walls stay closed to sugar because there is not enough insulin. The cell walls can also stay closed because the insulin that is produced by the pancreas cannot be used by the cells.

When sugar cannot enter the cells, the sugar in the bloodstream goes higher and higher. The sugar may start to spill out into the urine. As the blood sugar gets higher, it may cause the following symptoms to occur:

- fatigue (tired feeling)
- thirst
- passing urine more often
- hungry
- weight loss
- blurry vision
- sexual problems
- itching
- numbness or pain in fingers, toes, feet

Without sugar to burn for energy, the cells begin to burn fat. Fat is a fuel our body has stored for emergencies.

When fat is burned in diabetes, poisons are produced. These poisons are called *ketones*. When ketones build up in the body you are in danger of becoming very ill. Ketones are a signal that diabetes is out of control. (Chapter 4 will explain ketones in more detail.)

Not all people with diabetes have the symptoms listed above. In fact, many people find out they have diabetes during a routine visit to their doctor—their blood sugar test is high. Even if you have no symptoms of diabetes, the blood sugar level must still be controlled because high blood sugar can affect many body systems.

NEW TERMS FOR DIABETES DIAGNOSIS

There is a new classification system for the types of diabetes. Diabetes is no longer called adult onset or juvenile onset. The new terms are as follows:

Type I diabetes: Insulin dependent diabetes—this was known as brittle, ketosis-prone diabetes, juvenile onset, and juvenile diabetes.

Type II diabetes: Non-insulin dependent diabetes—there are two subdivisions: *nonobese* and *obese*. This was known as adult onset, maturity onset, ketosis-resistant diabetes, stable diabetes, or maturity-onset diabetes in youths.

Impaired Glucose Tolerance: Was known as latent, borderline, chemical, or asymptomatic diabetes.

Gestational diabetes: Increased blood sugar during pregnancy. This diabetes often improves soon after delivery.

Previous Abnormal Glucose Tolerance: Was known as prediabetes.

Potential Abnormal Glucose Tolerance: Was known as potential diabetes or prediabetes.

Evaluate Yourself 1

1. What is diabetes?

2. What are five symptoms of high blood sugar?

3. What is the normal range of blood sugar?

4. What factors make a person more likely to get diabetes?

5. Do all diabetics have symptoms of high blood sugar?

Answers to Evaluate Yourself 1

1. Diabetes is a life-long disease in which your body does not use food
   correctly.

2. Symptoms of high blood sugar are thirst, frequent urination, blurry
   vision, fatigue, pain or numbness in the fingers or toes, constant
   hunger, and/or weight loss.

3. Normal blood sugar is 70–110 mg%.

4. People are more likely to get diabetes if they have a family history of
   diabetes, if they are overweight, or if they are under stress. Older
   people are also more likely to get diabetes.

5. No, many people have no symptoms of diabetes.

URINE TESTING

If you have diabetes you will want to keep your blood sugar as close to
normal as you possibly can. Research today supports the fact that day-to-
day control of blood sugar may help delay, if not prevent, chronic complications of diabetes. You can test your urine for sugar each day. Urine
tests will help you control your blood sugar. Urine tests are one method of
checking the control of your diabetes. It is the least costly method.

In some people, urine testing does not accurately show the blood sugar
level. In this case, self blood sugar testing is suggested. Check with your
doctor or nurse about this.

Normal blood sugar is at a level of 70–110mg%. When the blood sugar is at this level there should be no sugar in the urine. In most people, the blood sugar must rise to 180mg% before it will spill into the urine. The *renal threshold* is the level at which sugar from the bloodstream begins to spill into the urine. The renal threshold varies greatly from person to person. One person may show sugar in the urine when the blood sugar level is 150mg%. Another person may not show sugar in the urine until the blood sugar reaches 300mg%.

For people with a high renal threshold (over 200mg%) urine testing may not be useful. Self blood sugar testing would be the best method for them.

As you can see, urine tests give you an idea about what your blood sugar is. The higher your blood sugar, the more sugar will spill into your urine. When you test your urine and keep a record of the tests, you will know when your blood sugar is too high.

These are some guidelines to follow for urine testing:

- Test your urine a number of times a day. Most diabetics taking insulin test before meals and at bedtime.
- Test urine recently made by your kidneys. Urine which has been held in your bladder for many hours may not give you the right test result. To test fresh urine (called a second-voided specimen), empty your bladder. Wait 15–30 minutes and go to the bathroom again. Test this new urine.
- Keep a record of your test results. Take this record to your doctor at your next appointment.
- If your urine tests show ½%, 1%, or 2% sugar, you should also test for ketones. Sugar and ketones in your urine are signs that your diabetes is out of control.

Follow these guidelines for calling your doctor:

- When sugar in the urine is ½%, 1%, or 2% for two days, call your doctor.
- When sugar *and* ketones are present in your urine for 24 hours, call your doctor.

There are many ways to test your urine for sugar and ketones. Ask your doctor or nurse which method would be best for you to use.

URINE TESTING EQUIPMENT

There are many types of urine testing methods for you to use. The color charts on the urine test method read "%" of sugar in the urine. The most common test methods are:

Tes-Tape®
Ketodiastix®, Diastix®, and Ketostix®
Clinistix®
Clinitest® and Acetest®
GK Chemstrip®

Tes-Tape®

Tes-Tape is the cheapest of the urine testing methods. There are about 100 tests in one dispenser of Tes-Tape. Tes-Tape only tests for sugar in the urine.

How to Use Tes-Tape®

1. Tear off about 1½ inches of tape.
2. Moisten the strip with urine and remove at once.
3. Use the second-hand of a watch or clock and time for one minute.
4. If the tape remains yellow, the urine is negative for sugar. If a color appears, compare the darkest area with the color chart on the dispenser. The range is ⅒%, ¼%, ½%, 2% or more.

Storage: Protect the tape from direct light, moisture, and heat. Store Tes-Tape in a cool, dry place. There is an expiration date printed on the Tes-Tape carton. The tape should not be used after this date or if the tape has turned brown.

Drawbacks: In the range from ⅒% to 2% it is hard to tell one color apart from the next. Ketones in the urine can affect Tes-Tape results. Ketones can make the urine sugar test read less than what it really is.

Ketodiastix®, Diastix®, and Ketostix®

Ketodiastix is the most expensive urine testing method. It tests for both sugar and ketones in the urine.

Diastix is next to Tes-Tape in being the least costly. Diastix tests only for sugar in the urine. Ketostix tests only for ketones in the urine.

How to use Ketodiastix®, Diastix®, and Ketostix®

1. Remove a strip and replace the cap.
2. Dip the end of the strip into the urine for two seconds and remove, or pass through the urine stream.
3. Tap edge of the strip against the side of the urine container or sink to remove excess urine.
4. *Immediately* after removing the strip from the container, begin

timing with a second-hand of a watch or clock.

5. Read the ketone test exactly fifteen seconds after dipping. If the pad stays beige, the test is negative for ketones. If a color appears, compare the color with the color chart on the bottle. The range is from trace to small, moderate, or large.

6. Read the sugar test exactly thirty seconds after dipping. If the pad remains blue, the urine is negative or 0% for sugar. If a color appears, compare the color with the color chart on the bottle. If it appears to be between two colors, choose the color that covers the most area in the center of the pad. The range is from $\frac{1}{10}$%, $\frac{1}{4}$%, $\frac{1}{2}$%, 1%, or 2%.

Storage: Protect the dipstick from direct light, heat, and humidity. Ketodiastix, Diastix, and Ketostix should be stored in a cool, dry place but not in the refrigerator. Keep the caps of the bottles on tight. Do not touch the pads with your fingers or with any other surface. There is an expiration date printed on each bottle. The "dipstick" should not be used after this date, or if the pads do not read negative before they are used.

Drawbacks: Dipsticks require exact timing. You cannot count the seconds without a watch or clock second hand. Ketones in the urine can affect the results of Ketodiastix and Diastix. Ketones can make the urine sugar test read less than what it really is.

GK Chemstrip®

GK Chemstrips test for both sugar and ketones in the urine.

How to Use the GK Chemstrip® method

1. Remove a strip from the container.
2. Dip the testing pad of the strip into the urine briefly (no longer than one (1) second). Make certain the testing pad is totally immersed.
3. Draw the edge of the strip along the edge of the container to remove the excess urine.
4. Wait exactly one (1) minute and compare the testing pad with the chart on the bottle. Normal and negative results for glucose may be recorded immediately. Ketone results may also be recorded now.
5. Glucose test results over $\frac{1}{10}$% on the chart should be read again after an additional four (4) minutes.

Drawbacks: Five (5) minutes timing is required for the results of urine sugars over normal.

Clinistix®

Clinistix tests only for sugar in the urine. Clinistix is useful for large-scale screening for diabetics.

How to Use the Clinistix® method

1. Remove a strip from the bottle and replace cap.
2. Dip end of the strip into the urine or pass it quickly through the urine stream.
3. Tap edge of the strip against the side of the urine container or sink it into the container to remove excess urine.
4. *Immediately* after removing the strip from the urine, begin timing with a second-hand of a watch or clock. Read the sugar test precisely ten seconds after removing the strip from the urine.
5. Compare the strip to the closest matching color block. If it remains pink, it is negative for sugar. The range is: small $\frac{1}{10}$%, medium $\frac{1}{4}$%, or large $\frac{3}{4}$%.

Storage: Do not touch the test area of the strip. Protect the dipstick from direct light, heat, and moisture. Clinistix should be stored in a cool, dry place but not in a refrigerator. There is an expiration date printed on each bottle. Dipsticks should not be used after this date or if the pads do not read negative before they are used.

Drawbacks: The range of sugar in the urine is small compared to other urine testing methods.

Clinitest® and Acetest®

Clinitest is the second most costly urine testing method. Clinitest tests only for sugar. Acetest tests only for ketones in the urine or blood.

How to Use the Clinitest® method

1. Take the dropper and put two drops of urine in the test tube to use the Clinitest two-drop method. If you are using the Clinitest five-drop method, put five drops of urine in the test tube.
2. Rinse the dropper. Place ten drops of water in the test tube.
3. Place one Clinitest tablet in the test tube.
4. Watch while the bubbling action takes place. Do not shake the test tube.
5. Wait fifteen seconds after the boiling stops. Shake the test tube gently.
6. Compare the tube's color with the color chart in the Clinitest kit. If

the tube is dark blue, it is negative or 0% sugar. The range is from ¼%, ½%, ¾%, 1%, or 2% for the five-drop method. If the color rapidly "passes through" green, tan, and orange to a dark greenish brown, record the result as over 2%. A different chart is used for the two-drop method.

How to Use the Acetest® tablets

1. Place one tablet on a clean surface.
2. Put one drop of urine on the tablet.
3. Wait for thirty seconds. Time with the second-hand of a watch or clock.
4. Compare the tablet color to the chart. If the tablet color remains the same or turns cream-colored, it is negative for ketones. The ranges are small, moderate, or large for amounts of ketones present.

Storage of Clinitest and Acetest tablets: Protect the tablets from moisture. Keep the bottles tightly closed. Store the tablets in a dry place. Keep them away from direct heat and sunlight. Do not use the Clinitest tablets that have turned dark blue. They have absorbed moisture and will give you wrong results.

Drawbacks: These tablets are toxic and corrosive. Keep them away from children or confused adults. Clinitest is harder to use. A dropper, test tube, tablets, and a cup for the urine is needed. The Clinitest method is affected by sugars other than glucose in the urine, aspirin taken in large doses, and high doses of antibiotics.

PLUSES TO PERCENTAGES

As of February 1, 1980, all urine test result charts were changed. Now, the result is read as percentages—% of sugar spill. Your urine test used to be read as pluses—+.

Before this date, a "1+" could mean ½%, or ⅒% of sugar. Each urine test method had its own values. Now, no matter what method you are using, your result is always a percent of the sugar spill.

Table 1-1 compares the common urine testing methods. The table compares each "+" of a sugar spill to a "%" of a sugar spill.

Table 1-1. Comparisons of common urine testing methods using "%" and "+."

Urine Test Method	1/10%	1/4%	1/2%	3/4%	1%	2%	Over 2%
Clinitest	Neg.	Trace	1+	2+	3+	4+	5+
Diastix	Trace	1+	2+		3+	4+	
Tes-Tape	1+	2+	3+				
Clinistix	-------Light-------Medium--------------Dark-------------						
GK Chemstrip	1+	2+			3+	4+	

SELF BLOOD SUGAR TESTING

Urine tests tell you only when your blood sugar is high. Self blood sugar testing tells you a specific blood-sugar reading. This is the reason some people are replacing urine testing with self blood sugar testing. It may also be called self glucose testing. It is the most accurate test method at the present time.

Normal blood sugar is 70–110mg%. A safe range for you is 70–140mg%. The normal pre-meal level for adults is about 90mg%.

In most people, blood sugar must rise to 180mg% before it spills over into the urine. This is called the *renal threshold*. Thus, even a 1/10% or a trace reading could mean the blood sugar is already over 180mg%. If a person's renal threshold is even higher, such as 200mg%, urine test results can seem "low" even when the blood sugar is far above the safe range of 70–140mg%. Many factors can change the renal threshold. These factors can raise or lower the level at which sugar is spilled into the urine. For instance, the renal threshold may be lowered by exercise, pregnancy, or fever. Some of the factors raising the renal threshold include chronic high blood sugar, old age, kidney disease, or heart failure.

There is also a lag time between blood sugar rise and the spill of sugar into the urine. This may vary from time to time. Your blood sugar may be high but you may not spill sugar into your urine for 20 minutes to two hours later. Your urine test can read negative even though your blood sugar is rising.

Self blood sugar testing tells you exactly what your blood sugar is at any given time. For this reason, many people prefer this method of monitoring their control over urine testing. The major disadvantage of self blood sugar testing is the expense. Strips alone are the least expensive method. It is possible to obtain accurate results with the use of the test strips alone. There are two strips on the market: bG Chemstrip®

manufactured by Biodynamic, and Visidex® manufactured by Ames. Each strip uses a drop of blood on a reagent pad. Use of a machine for a precise digital readout will increase the cost. There are a variety of machines available to use in self testing of blood sugars. Talk to your doctor or diabetes educator about the use of a machine. They can explain types, costs, and other facts.

Blood sugar testing is usually recommended four times a day before meals and bedtime just as it is for urine testing. Blood sugar testing can also be done to detect low blood sugars. You can test again after treating low blood sugar to measure the rise in your blood sugar. Many people use self blood sugar testing to determine how much exercise lowers their blood sugars.

Follow these guidelines for calling your doctor:

- If your blood sugar is over 240mg%, start testing your urine for ketones. Call if there are ketones present for 24 hours.
- When your blood sugar is over 240mg% for two days.

Blood Testing Equipment

The first step in self blood sugar testing is drawing a drop of blood from a finger. After proper handwashing, allow your hands to dry. Next, take a special needle and make a very tiny prick. The best place to prick is on the sides of the finger pads. The nerves (pain sensors) tend to be on the part of your finger that makes a fingerprint. If you use the sides you will have the least amount of discomfort. A large drop of blood can be squeezed from a very small hole. Drop the sample onto the test strip and measure.

Discuss the various machines and test strips available for self blood sugar testing with your nurse or doctor. Those who should perform self blood sugar monitoring include:

1. pregnant diabetics
2. diabetics on insulin pumps
3. labile diabetics
4. diabetics with complications, especially of the small blood vessels
5. diabetics with an altered renal threshold
6. all diabetic children under five years of age
7. diabetics with these special situations:
   a. renal dialysis
   b. those on cortisone
   c. nighttime insulin reactions
   d. athletic competition

Evaluate Yourself 2

1. Why do you need to test your urine or blood and record the results?

2. What time of day should you test your urine or blood?

3. What is a second-voided specimen?

4. When should you call your doctor about your urine or blood test results?

Answers to Evaluate Yourself 2

1. Testing your urine or blood and keeping a record of the tests gives you an idea of how well your diabetes is controlled.
2. You should test your urine or blood four times a day, before meals and bedtime.
3. A second-voided specimen is a sample of urine you collect by first emptying your bladder. In 15–30 minutes go to the bathroom again and test this new urine.
4. Call the doctor after two days if your urine sugar is ½%, 1%, or 2%. Call the doctor in one day if your urine tests are ½%, 1%, or 2% with ketones. Call your doctor after two days if your blood tests are over 240mg%. Call your doctor if your blood sugar is over 240mg%, and ketones are present for 24 hours.

2

Keeping In Balance

DIABETES CONTROL

If you have diabetes you and your doctor will choose the control method which is best for you. There are three methods of control:

1. The diabetic diet and exercise;
2. The diabetic diet, exercise, and oral hypoglycemic pills;
3. The diabetic diet, exercise, and insulin injections.

The diabetic diet and an exercise program are the basis of control for everyone with diabetes.

Remember the goals of diabetes control:

- To keep the blood sugar as close to the normal range as you can. Discuss this with your doctor. Ask your doctor what your blood sugar should be. He or she may want you to visit on a regular schedule so that he or she can check your blood sugar. Your doctor will also want you to test your urine or blood for sugar on a daily basis. This will give you an idea of what your blood sugar is from day to day.
- To feel well, and free, of the symptoms of uncontrolled diabetes.
- To avoid or delay the complications of diabetes.

We will take a closer look at the control methods after your evaluation quiz.

Evaluate Yourself 1

1. Why is it important to control diabetes?

2. What are three methods to control diabetes?

3. Which method do you use to control your blood sugar?

Answers to Evaluate Yourself 1

1. It is important to control diabetes so that you will keep your blood sugar as close to normal as possible, feel well, and avoid or delay the complications of diabetes.
2. Three methods of controlling diabetes are:
   a. diet and exercise
   b. diet, exercise, and oral hypoglycemics
   c. diet, exercise, and insulin
3. I control my diabetes with _____

   _____

   _____

CONTROL:
YOU ARE WHAT YOU EAT

The food that you eat and drink is the most important, and often the most difficult, part of diabetes treatment. You may have to alter your present eating style. You and your dietitian or nutritionist will design your meal plan. Both of you will take into account your present food intake and its nutritional content, your lifestyle (social, ethnic, religious, economic, and work), activity level, and medications that you take.

There are three reasons why the diabetic meal plan is so important:

- You can control your blood sugar
- You can control your weight
- You will eat well-balanced meals

Most of the food that you or a non-diabetic person eats or drinks can be changed into blood sugar. This sugar is called *glucose*. Glucose travels in your blood. It gives you energy. You need glucose to keep going every day. You must have a balance between sugar from the food that you eat and the insulin that you get from your pancreas or your injection or with the help of the oral hypoglycemic pills.

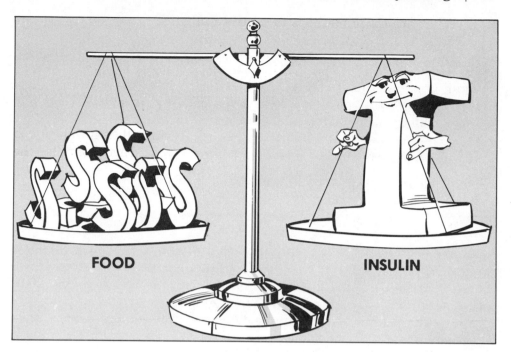

FOOD   INSULIN

You can control your blood sugar in these ways:

- Do not eat concentrated sweets on a regular or frequent basis. These foods provide more sugar than your body is able to use. Sugar will make your blood sugar go very high, very fast. Some of these sweets include sugar, honey, syrup, candy, jellies, sweetened fruits and fruit drinks, pie, pastry, sweet rolls, and sweetened pop, soft drinks, or soda. Sometimes, some of these high sugar foods may be a part of your meal plan. There are also times when you may choose to include them in a meal or snack. You can discuss how and when to include these foods with your dietitian.
- Control the amount of the other foods that you eat. This includes milk, vegetables, fruits, starches, meats, and fat.

Your diet is also important because you need to control your weight. Your body functions and feels best at your ideal body weight. This is how you figure out your ideal body weight:

Males: If you are 5 feet tall, you should weigh 106 pounds.
           Add 6 pounds for each extra inch.

Females: If you are 5 feet tall, you should weigh 100 pounds.
           Add 5 pounds for each extra inch.

Besides height, your bone structure affects your weight. If you have small bones and are 5 feet tall, you will weigh less than a person who has large bones, who is also 5 feet tall.

Subtract 10% if you are small boned. Add 10% if you are large boned. The figures are not altered if you are medium boned.

If you are under 5 foot 4 inches tall, you are:

small boned if your wrist is less than 5½ inches,
medium boned if your wrist is between 5½ to 5¾ inches,
large boned if your wrist is larger than 5¾ inches.

If you are 5 foot 4 inches or taller, you are:

small boned if your wrist is less than 6¼ inches,
medium boned if your wrist is between 6¼ to 6½ inches,
large boned is your wrist is larger than 6½ inches.

A goal of your diet is to help you reach and maintain your ideal body weight. You can do this by changing your meal plan to meet your needs. Some of the factors that affect your needs are your age, your sex, your present weight, your activity level, and your work schedule.

Your calorie level depends on whether you weigh more or less than what you should. This depends on whether you are at your ideal body weight. You and your doctor or a dietitian will decide on your calorie level.

A *calorie* is a measure of the energy value of food. If you eat more calories than you use up, you will gain weight. If you eat fewer calories than you burn up, you will lose weight. If you eat 100 extra calories a day, you will gain 10 pounds of fat in one year.

Extra weight is a problem in many adults with diabetes. This makes your diet doubly important—for weight loss as well as control of your blood sugar.

Last, your diet is a well-balanced eating plan. Your diet gives you the right amounts of protein, fat, carbohydrate, minerals, vitamins, and water. These are the nutrients that help your body to grow, to repair itself, and to provide a sense of well-being. Each of these "nutrients" has its own function within the body. Three of these nutrients have calories and affect your blood sugar: carbohydrate, protein, and fat. Vitamins, minerals, and water do *not* affect your blood sugar, nor do they provide calories.

Carbohydrate includes all sugars and starches. Most of the time, *all of the carbohydrate that you eat in food breaks down into blood sugar.* Carbohydrate is your main source of energy. You must eat some carbohydrate everyday. Milk, vegetables, fruits, breads and cereals, and sugar are examples of foods that contain carbohydrate.

A *gram* is a unit of weight in the metric system. A gram is ¹⁄₂₈ of an ounce. As a guideline, a paperclip weighs one gram. Twenty-eight grams equals one ounce. A lot of the time we round this figure off to 30 grams.

When you eat one gram of carbohydrate, you produce four calories.

1 gram carbohydrate
equals
4 calories

Protein is used to build and repair your body. Of the protein that you eat in food, about 58 percent can break down to blood sugar most of the time. The best sources of protein are meat, fish, eggs, poultry, and dairy products. When you eat one gram of protein, you produce four calories.

1 gram protein
equals
4 calories

Fat is your stored energy and also adds flavor and variety to your diet. Most of the time, ten percent of the fat that you eat in food can break down to blood sugar. Butter, margarine, oils, cream, nuts, and whole milk are fat sources. Fat is the most concentrated source of calories. Fat has a very small effect on your blood sugar. When you eat one gram of fat, you produce nine calories.

1 gram fat
equals
9 calories

Evaluate Yourself 2

1. Why is a nutritious diet important to you? _____, _____, and _____.

2. What does a lot of sugar in food do to your blood sugar?

3. What are eight foods that contain a large amount of sugar?

4. How much does carbohydrate (CHO) affect your blood sugar?

5. What percentage of protein affects your blood sugar?

6. What percentage of fat affects your blood sugar?

7. What is your ideal body weight?

8. What is one gram equal to in nonmetric terms?

9. How many calories are there in one gram of carbohydrate?

10. How many calories are there in one gram of protein?

11. How many calories are there in one gram of fat?

12. How many calories are there in water?

13. How many calories are there in vitamins and minerals?

14. Do vitamins and minerals affect your blood sugar?

Answers to Evaluate Yourself 2

1. control your blood sugar
   control your weight
   help you eat well-balanced meals & snacks.
2. Sugar makes the blood sugar level go high very fast.
3. See your sugar list.
4. 100 percent
5. 58 percent
6. 10 percent
7. My ideal body weight is _____.
8. ⅟₂₈ of an ounce.
9. 4 calories per 1 gram of carbohydrate
10. 4 calories per 1 gram of protein
11. 9 calories per 1 gram of fat
12. No calories in water
13. No calories in vitamins and minerals
14. Vitamins and minerals do *not* affect your blood sugar.

EXERCISE

Exercise and good eating habits are the cornerstones of diabetes control!

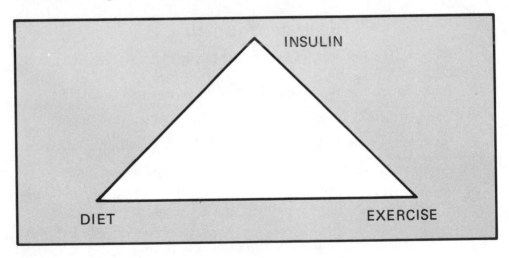

Here are some benefits that exercise has for you.

1. Strengthens the heart and other muscles.
2. Helps you to reach and maintain your ideal weight.
3. Keeps your body joints flexible.
4. Helps keep your blood vessels elastic.
5. Improves the blood flow in your body.

6. Relieves tension.
7. Provides a general feeling of better health and joy.
8. Feeling better means an improved self-concept.
9. Exercise burns blood sugar at a faster rate. This is the way it decreases your blood sugar. This decreases the amount of insulin your body needs. You need to take smaller amounts of insulin if you exercise regularly.

Every person can exercise in some way. If you have not been involved in a routine exercise program, discuss your diabetes control, precautions, side effects, and program with your doctor and/or an exercise specialist. Your doctor might want you to have a physical exam, an ECG (electrocardiogram), or a stress test. These tests will help define your personal activity program.

Here are some ways to enjoy your exercise program more.

- Exercise at about the same time each day to help you keep your insulin and food intake stable.
- Exercise that is performed daily will help you control your blood sugar. If you cannot do it daily, then exercise at least three times a week.
- Ask someone else to exercise with you. It is more fun. The other person must know that you have diabetes, so that they can deal with any problems that might come up.
- Wear shoes that fit you well. You want to prevent problems, like blisters.
- Take extra care with an injury.
- Carry small change. You may need it to buy food from a vending machine or to make a phone call.
- Bring extra food on a day long trip. You may find it helpful to eat six small meals a day to have a more frequent source of energy.
- Before you exercise, eat a small serving of food low in fat. You could eat fruit, crackers, and cereals. Foods high in fat will stay in your stomach longer. These foods may cause some discomfort.
- Drink plenty of fluids like water. You do not want to become dehydrated from exercising.
- Exercise after you eat. This is the best time. Your blood sugar is starting to increase about 15 to 30 minutes after your meal.

If you take insulin or oral pills:

- Do not inject insulin into a part of the body you will be exercising. This will cause insulin to be used at a faster than normal rate. You could have an insulin reaction. Use a non-exercised area for insulin injection. For instance, when you walk or run, use your abdomen for injection. Your goal is to maintain the balance between food and insulin while you exercise.

- You can keep your insulin dose the same and eat more food. Or, you can reduce your dose and eat the same amount of food. It is easier to alter your food intake. You may change your planned activity at the last minute. Discuss a decrease in your insulin dose with your doctor.

- You must plan a snack if you prefer to exercise before a meal or on an empty stomach. There are as many kinds of snacks as there are foods. You may have to test how certain foods affect your blood sugar during and after exercise. For instance,
  —Before each hour of exercise, you can eat one fruit or bread-starch exchange.
  —Before every two hours of activity you can eat:
    - ½ sandwich, or
    - 6 crackers and two slices of cheese, or
    - one piece of toast and ½ cup of milk, or
    - 6 crackers and 2 tablespoons of peanut butter

This food will prevent an insulin reaction. See the chapter on insulin reactions.

- Always carry some form of sugar with you. You may have a low blood sugar reaction (insulin reaction or hypoglycemic reaction).

- You can use self blood sugar testing to help you assess your body's need for insulin and food. The best time to test is before and after your exercise period.

- Do not exercise when your blood sugar is low. Also, do not begin to exercise when your insulin is reaching its peak effect.

- You may have to eat more than usual after you have stopped your activity. Exercise has a long-lasting effect. You can become hypoglycemic or your blood sugar can fall many hours after you finish your activity.

What are the elements of an exercise program?

- *Flexibility to increase the range of motion of your joints*. You can stretch to warm up. Do a long slow stretch, but do not bounce. Ask an exercise specialist to show you exercises that will increase your flexibility.

- *Activities to increase the strength of your muscles*. You want your muscles to exert a force over and over or to hold a certain position. Curl ups will strengthen the stomach muscles. Side leg lifts will strengthen the thighs. Have an exercise specialist show you how to increase your muscle strength.

- *Relaxation can release excess tension in your muscles.* When you take deep breaths your muscles begin to relax.
- *Cardiovascular endurance or aerobic activity.* These activities cause an increase in oxygen need. You will use many muscles over a long period of time. Your blood system and heart is stressed by this activity. You can measure the stress on your heart and lungs by checking your pulse rate. You can increase your endurance level by walking fast, running, jogging, swimming, bicycling, dancing, and other forms of activity.

Your Exercise Program

These guidelines are for people who do not have any health problems. Consult with your doctor before you begin a program.

- Know your resting pulse rate. Someone may have to help you feel your pulse the first time. Take your pulse after you sit quietly for a few minutes. Count the beats for ten seconds. Multiply by six to get your 60 second rate.

- Know your target heart rate before you start. You want to know how intense your activity can be. The faster the pulse rate, the more intense your activity. Your age is also taken into account. These are some factors used in considering heart rate:
  - The maximum heart rate is 220 beats per minute.
  - Subtract your age from the maximum heart rate.
  - Figure out your maximum range. It will be 50, 60, 70, or 85%. Multiply this percent by the above figure (220) to get your range for one minute. Your doctor or exercise specialist can also tell you what level to use. Divide by six to know your ten second range. The maximum range is 50 percent if you have not been active. The maximum range for a conditioned athlete is 85 percent.
  - Do not exceed your maximum range.

Table 2-1 shows the ten second and 60 second heart rates that take your age into account. Find your age on this table. Read across to find your range.

Table 2-1. Maximum Heart Rate.

Age	60 SECOND RANGE			10 SECOND RANGE		
	60% maximum	70% maximum	85% maximum	60% maximum	70% maximum	85% maximum
25–26	117	136	116	20	22	27
27–28	116	135	164	19	22	27
29	115	134	162	19	22	26
30–31	114	133	161	19	22	26
32–33	113	132	160	19	22	26
34	112	130	158	19	22	26
35–36	111	129	157	19	22	26
37–38	110	128	155	18	21	25
39	109	127	154	18	21	25
40–41	108	126	153	18	21	25
42–43	107	125	151	18	21	25
44	106	123	150	18	21	25
45	105	122	149	18	21	25
50	102	119	145	18	21	25
55	99	116	140	17	19	23

When you begin an exercise program, start slowly! Increase the length of your activity program to about 30—40 minutes per day with a warm-up and cool-down over a period of four to six weeks.

Do not increase the intensity, how *hard* you are working, and the duration, how *long* you are working, at the same time. If you increase the intensity, do not increase the duration. If you increase the duration, do not increase the intensity. In order to increase your aerobic endurance, you need to exercise a minimum of three times a week. Exercise every other day, not three days in a row so that you retain the benefits of your activity. For most noncompetitive athletes, it is a good idea not to do aerobic activity more than five times a week. When you exercise more than five times a week you may have injuries. Check with your exercise specialist or doctor to help you decide the intensity and duration of your exercise program.

Do not exercise when you have:

- Ketones in your urine
- Diabetes that is out of control. When your blood sugar is already elevated, exercise will only cause a greater rise in your blood sugar. Omit exercise until your diabetes is controlled.
- Chest pain or angina
- Pain in your shoulders or arms
- Severe shortness of breath.

Do not exercise if you have:

- Neuropathy—do not jog. You can swim or ride a bike.
- Hypertension—do not do isometric exercises.

If you have had a myocardial infarction (MI) discuss your program with your doctor.

There are some drugs that may have adverse effects if you exercise while using them. Discuss the adverse effect any drugs you are taking may have with your doctor or exercise specialist.

There are many forms of exercise from walking to team sports. Choose one that is fun for you. ENJOY!

Evaluate Yourself 3

1. List four benefits of exercise.

2. Does exercise increase or decrease blood sugar?

3. If you take oral pills or insulin, what should you do before exercising?

4. Where do you inject your insulin when you exercise?

5. At what time of day should you exercise?

6. What are the four elements of an exercise program?

7. What is your target heart rate?

8. How often should you exercise?

9. How long should your exercise program last?

10. When must you stop your exercise program?

11. Which exercise program can you do?

Answers to Evaluate Yourself 3

1. Exercise strengthens the heart and other muscles. It helps you reach and maintain your ideal weight. Exercise keeps body joints

flexible and keeps blood vessels elastic. It improves the blood flow in your body, and relieves tension. Exercise provides a general feeling of better health—joy! Feeling better means an improved self-concept. Exercise also decreases blood sugar. /

2. Exercise *decreases* blood sugar.

3. Eat! You may choose one fruit or bread-starch exchange for every hour of exercise. You could eat ½ sandwich, or six crackers and two slices of cheese, or one piece of toast and ½ glass of milk, or six crackers and two tablespoons of peanut butter for every two hours of exercise.

4. Inject insulin in an area you do not use during your activity.

5. Exercise after you eat.

6. Four elements of an exercise program are *joint flexibility, muscle strength, body relaxation,* and *cardiovascular endurance.*

7. My target heart rate is _____.

8. Exercise every day or a minimum of three times a week.

9. Exercise for 30–40 minutes at a time.

10. If you experience chest, shoulder, or arm pain, or shortness of breath. Do not jog if you have neuropathy.

11. My daily exercise program is _____

ORAL HYPOGLYCEMIC PILLS

Hypoglycemic pills are taken by mouth to lower blood sugar. Hypoglycemic pills are not insulin. These pills lower the blood sugar by helping the pancreas produce more insulin. These pills cannot be taken by all diabetics. Normally, people who get diabetes before age 30 cannot control their blood sugar with pills. Many other diabetics are not helped by the pills and must use insulin injections, diet, and exercise to control their blood sugar. You and your doctor will decide if pills are a safe way for you to control your diabetes. If you do take a hypoglycemic pill, you should know these facts:

- The diabetic diet is still a vital part of control. Hypoglycemic pills do not cure diabetes. If you do not follow your diet, the pills will not help you.

- Hypoglycemic pills lower blood sugar. This means that you must eat meals and snacks on time to avoid low blood sugar reactions.

- Take your pills as prescribed by your doctor. Try to take the pills at the same time each day.

- Know the name of your pill and carry or wear identification which states you are a diabetic and take _____ (your pill). The

types of hypoglycemic pills are listed below:
Orinase®
Diabenese®
Tolinase®
Dymelor®

- Do not take extra pills unless your doctor tells you to. Avoid using over-the-counter medicines (such as cough drops, cough syrups, and cold tablets) without asking your doctor first. Some of these medicines can affect your blood sugar.
- When extra stress is placed on your body by surgery, accident, illness or emotions, your doctor may decide that you need insulin injections to control your blood sugar.
- A prescription is required from your doctor for hypoglycemic pills.

Evaluate Yourself 4

1. How do hypoglycemic pills lower the blood sugar?

2. What is the name of the oral hypoglycemic pill you take?

3. What time of the day do you take your pill(s), and what is the dose you take?

Answers to Evaluate Yourself 4

1. The hypoglycemic pills lower blood sugar by stimulating the pancreas to produce more insulin.
2. The hypoglycemic pill I take is _____ .
3. I take my hypoglycemic pill(s) at _____ .
   My hypoglycemic pills are _____ (dose).

INSULIN

When Type II diabetes cannot be controlled by diet alone or by diet and hypoglycemic pills, your doctor may prescribe insulin. Your doctor will always prescribe insulin if you have Type I diabetes. Insulin is needed in your bloodstream to help sugar enter your cells. Insulin cannot be taken by mouth. Insulin is a protein which our bodies would destroy before it could enter the bloodstream. Insulin must be given with a needle and syringe into the fatty tissue under the skin. Tiny blood vessels found under the skin slowly absorb insulin into the bloodstream.

Types of Insulin

If you take insulin, you should know which type you take and how it acts on your body to lower blood sugar. The types of insulin can be put into four groups: short-acting insulin, short and intermediate-acting combination, intermediate-acting insulin, and long-acting insulin. Each group is discussed below.

Short-acting Insulins: Regular®, Semilente®, Actrapid®, and Velosulin®

Short-acting insulins start to work quickly. They last for 8–12 hours in the body. Their peak action (the time of day at which they lower the blood sugar the most) is about 2–5 hours after injecting.

Regular insulin is often used mixed with an intermediate-acting insulin. Regular insulin is also used when a diabetic is under stress due to illness or surgery and needs close control of blood sugars with frequent injections.

Intermediate-acting Insulins: NPH®, Lente®, Monotard®, Lentard®, Insulatard®, and Semitard®

Intermediate-acting insulins take effect within two hours of injection. They work best 8–12 hours after injecting and most last for 18–24 hours in the body. Semitard does not last as long as the rest of these insulins. Semitard will last about 16 hours in the body. The intermediate-acting insulins should be taken about one-half hour before eating breakfast unless your doctor gives you other instructions.

Short and Intermediate-acting Combination Insulin: Mixtard®

This is a combination type of insulin. Mixtard starts to work quickly like the short-acting insulins. It lasts for 24 hours in the body like the intermediate insulin. The peak action is in 4–8 hours.

Long-acting Insulins: PZI®, Ultralente®, Ultratard®

The long-acting insulins work for a longer time in your body. But, there is a greater danger in that your blood sugar will drop too low during the early morning hours when these insulins are used.

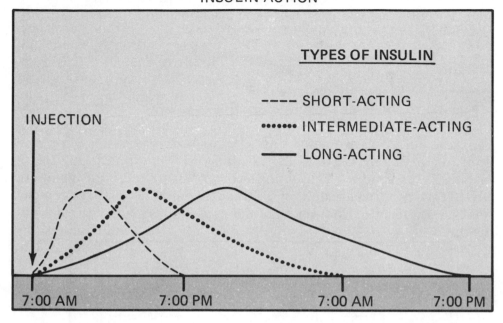

Figure 2–3 shows the action of the types of insulin mentioned above.

Concentration of Insulin

There are two concentrations of insulin that people can use: U-40 and U-100. Concentration refers to the number of units of insulin per cubic centimeter. As an example, U-40 means that in one cubic centimeter there are 40 units of insulin. Figure 2-4 shows U-40 and U-100 insulin. As you can see, U-100 insulin has more dots in the same amount of space and therefore is more concentrated.

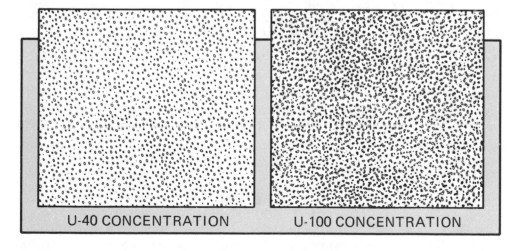

Most diabetics today use U-100 insulin. In a few years U-100 may be the only concentration you can buy. If you are now using U-40 insulin you can change to U-100 easily:

- buy U-100 insulin (the same type you are taking—NPH, Lente, or other insulin),
- buy U-100 insulin syringes, and
- measure the same amount of insulin as always.

For example, if you are now using 20 units of U-40 Lente insulin and want to start using U-100 Lente insulin, you would buy U-100 Lente insulin, U-100 insulin syringes, and measure 20 units of U-100 insulin in a U-100 syringe. Twenty units of U-40 and 20 units of U-100 will give the same dose of insulin. However, the amount of fluid is more with the U-40 insulin.

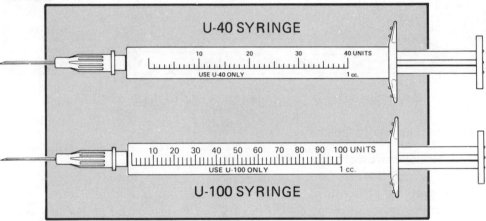

If you have questions about U-100 insulin, ask your doctor, nurse, or pharmacist for help.

STORING INSULIN

You should not let your insulin get too hot or too cold. Keep the bottle you are using at room temperature (68–80 degrees Fahrenheit). It is important that the insulin you inject be at room temperature. Cold insulin can cause depressions to form in the skin. Extra bottles of insulin should be refrigerated. If your insulin freezes or is exposed to temperatures above 120 degrees, it should not be used. Check your insulin bottle for the expiration date. Do not use the insulin after this date.

GIVING INSULIN

Insulin is measured in units. Your doctor will tell you how many units to take each day. Do not change the number of units unless your doctor tells you how to do so. Some diabetics need two injections or more daily to control their blood sugar. Your doctor will decide if this is needed in your case. *Never* give yourself extra insulin unless you are told how to do so by your doctor.

If you are now learning to give yourself insulin, ask your nurse to show you how. You will want to practice measuring and giving yourself insulin several times with your nurse watching you. You and your nurse want to be sure you can safely give yourself insulin at home. A family member should also learn to give you your insulin. The following are written instructions for giving insulin.

HOW TO GIVE SINGLE DOSES OF INSULIN

1. Wash your hands.
2. Turn the bottle upside down.
3. Roll the bottle between your hands to insure mixing of the insulin.
4. Wipe off the top of the bottle with cotton and alcohol or an alcohol wipe.
5. Measure _____ units of air. The bottle is airtight. (The air is needed to displace insulin to be withdrawn later.)
6. Push the needle through the rubber seal and push air into the bottle.
7. Turn the bottle upside down.
8. Pull the plunger halfway down the syringe.
9. Hold the bottle up straight and inject insulin back into the bottle to get rid of any air bubbles.
10. Measure _____ units of insulin. Look again for air bubbles.
11. Pull the bottle off the needle.
12. Cover the needle with the cap it was packaged in. Lay the syringe down.
13. Wipe your skin with cotton and alcohol or an alcohol wipe.
14. Spread your fingers approximately 3 inches apart and pinch your skin gently.
15. Pick up the syringe like a pencil or a dart.
16. Insert the needle at a 90° angle if you are of normal weight or over. If you are underweight, use a 45° angle to insert the needle.
17. Push down on the syringe plunger to inject the insulin.
18. Withdraw the needle and place an alcohol wipe over the area.
19. Wipe your skin gently.

WHERE TO GIVE INSULIN

Insulin should be given in areas inside the dotted lines. Avoid areas within an inch of the navel and scars. When an injection is given, write the date next to the number listed on the left side of this sheet. Do not give an injection in that site for at least one month.

Site	Date	Site	Date
1		24	
2		25	
3		26	
4		27	
5		28	
6		29	
7		30	
8		31	
9		32	
10		33	
11		34	
12		35	
13		36	
14		37	
15		38	
16		39	
17		40	
18		41	
19		42	
20		43	
21		44	
22		45	
23		46	

HOW TO GIVE MIXED DOSES OF INSULIN
(Intermediate plus short-acting)

1. Wash your hands and assemble the things you will need for your injection.

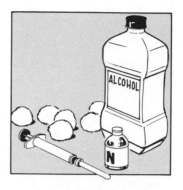

2. Turn the bottle upside down.

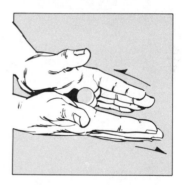

3. Roll the bottle between your hands to insure the mixing of the insulin.

4. Wipe off the bottle with cotton and alcohol or an alcohol wipe.

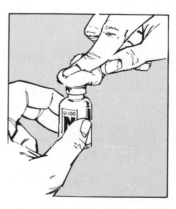

5. Measure _____ units of air for intermediate type insulin.

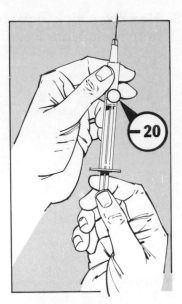

6. Push the needle through the rubber seal and inject air into the intermediate type bottle.

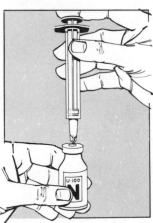

7. Withdraw the needle. The syringe is now empty.

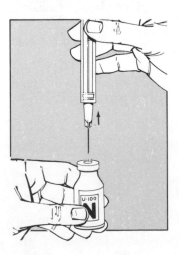

8. Measure _____ units of air (for regular or Semilente insulin).

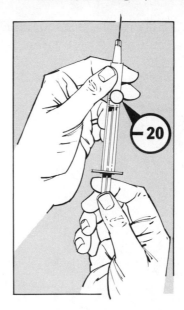

9. Push the needle through the rubber seal and inject air into the short-acting bottle.

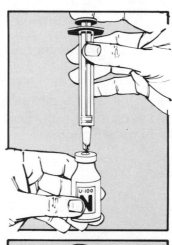

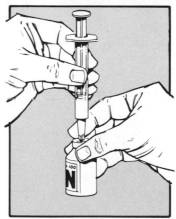

10. Turn the bottle upside down.

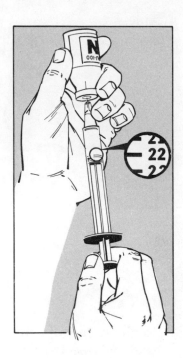

11. Pull the plunger half-way down the syringe.

12. Hold the bottle upright and inject insulin back into the bottle to get rid of any air bubbles.

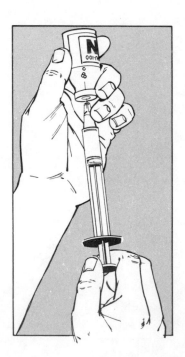

13. Measure _____ units of regular insulin. Look again for air bubbles.

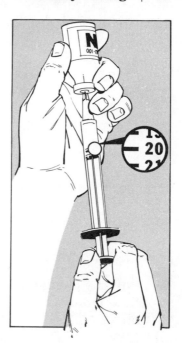

14. Carefully withdraw the needle.

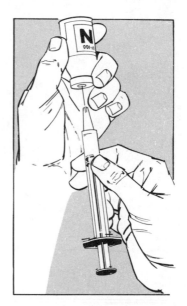

15. Turn the intermediate insulin bottle upside down and reinsert the needle.

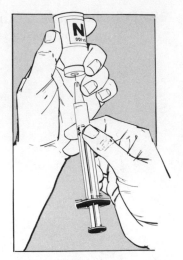

16. Pull the plunger slowly back to the total amount of _____ units: _____ plus _____ .

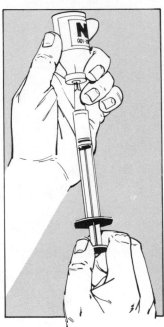

17. Pull the bottle off the needle.

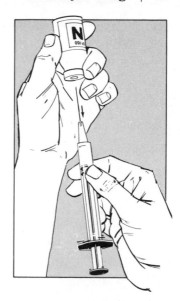

18. Cover the needle with the cap it was packaged in.

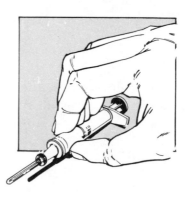

19. Wipe your skin with cotton and alcohol or an alcohol wipe.

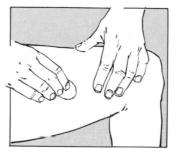

20. Spread your fingers approximately 3 inches apart.
21. Pick up the syringe like a dart.

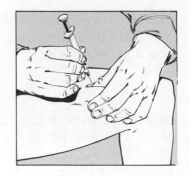

22. Insert the needle at a 90 degree angle if you are of normal weight or over. (If you are underweight, insert the needle at a 45 degree angle.)

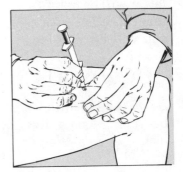

23. Push down on the syringe plunger to inject the insulin.

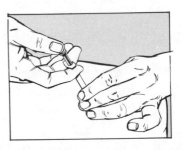

24. Withdraw the needle and place an alcohol wipe over the area.

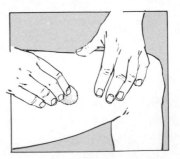

25. Wipe your skin gently.

Glass syringes should be stored in alcohol. Once a week they must be sterilized by boiling them. Ask your nurse for instructions if you want to use a glass syringe.

TRAVELING

When you go on a trip, always take extra insulin and syringes. Carry them with you. Do not put them in your luggage. If you are traveling out of the United States, take a letter from your doctor stating that you are a diabetic and require insulin. If you get ill or need to buy insulin, this letter will be helpful. In most states you do not need a doctor's order to buy insulin. It is a good practice to carry a written letter from your doctor if you will be on a long trip away from home.

HOW YOU CONTROL YOUR BLOOD SUGAR

If you take insulin you should know that you control your blood sugar by balancing food and exercise with your insulin. When a person does not have diabetes, the pancreas sends out just the right amount of insulin to balance food and exercise. When a person does not eat as much, less insulin is made. But, when you inject a certain amount of insulin each day, you must also eat a certain amount of food each day.

Here are some rules to help you keep "in balance."

- Take your insulin at about the same time each day.
- Eat your meals and snacks on time.
- Follow your meal plan and eat the same amount of food each day.
- Know when your insulin peaks.

No one lives on the same schedule day after day. Sometimes you will need to allow for changes in your mealtimes. Chapter Three, Insulin Reactions, will tell you how to do this safely.

PORTABLE INSULIN PUMPS

In the on-going search to maintain normal blood sugar, the insulin pump was developed. Similar in action to a real pancreas, the pump steadily puts out insulin at a low rate between meals. The pump delivers insulin at a higher rate just before meals. This higher dose before meals handles the added sugar obtained from eating. As a result, blood sugar can be maintained at almost normal ranges throughout the day and night.

Self-testing of blood sugar is essential when using an insulin pump. (See p. 13) The result of blood tests determine the rate of insulin given.

There are many different types of insulin pumps available. The average pump weighs about 10–13 ounces. These pumps can easily be worn on your belt.

The pumps use a portable syringe. This syringe can be manually operated or connected to a microcomputer to regulate insulin flow. The syringe is connected to a catheter (small tube). The catheter has a small needle at its end. This needle is inserted under the skin (usually in the abdomen) and taped down. The placement of the needle is changed every 2–5 days. The insulin pump can easily be removed for vigorous exercising, sexual activity, bathing or other similar activities. Regular insulin is the type used with an insulin pump.

Using an insulin pump allows for more flexibility with meals. Although you may delay your meal because you don't give the extra insulin until eating, you must still maintain a proper diet. Using excess food will result in a weight gain. This will make diabetes more difficult to control.

You must be carefully followed by your doctor when you use an insulin pump. Before starting on the pump you will need instruction by your doctor or diabetes educator.

Advantages of insulin pumps:

- sense of well-being
- allows participation in normal activities

Diabetic candidates for pump use:

- pregnant diabetics
- labile diabetics
- diabetics with complications
- any insulin-dependent diabetic who wants to obtain good blood sugar control.

Disadvantage of pump use:

- Worn externally

There is some research that indicates four separate doses of insulin per day can achieve results similiar to the insulin pump. If one objects to multiple needle injections, a jet injector may be available for use. Talk with your doctor or nurse about how to obtain this device.

Evaluate Yourself 5

1. What is the name and concentration of your insulin?

2. How many units do you take?

3. When should you take your insulin?

4. When does your insulin peak (work the hardest)?

5. Where are good places on the body to inject insulin?

6. Should the bottle of insulin you use be stored at room temperature or stored in the refrigerator?

Answers to Evaluate Yourself 5

1. The insulin I take is _____.
2. I take _____ units of _____ insulin.
3. I should take my insulin at _____.
4. My insulin peaks at _____.
5. Insulin should be given in many different areas of the body. You can use the back of the arms, thighs, abdomen, and buttocks. (See the figure on page 34)
6. The insulin you are using should be kept at room temperature.

3

Insulin Reactions

HYPOGLYCEMIA

People who take insulin or pills to control diabetes may have insulin reactions. Reactions happen when there is not enough sugar in your blood, or when there is a sudden drop in your blood sugar. A reaction may occur if:

- you do not eat enough food,
- you eat your meals and snacks late,
- you exercise without eating extra food, or
- you take too much insulin or too many pills.

There are other names for insulin reactions. They include low blood sugar, *hypoglycemia,* and insulin shock.

If you are on insulin or pills, you and your family or friends must know the early signs of a reaction. You must treat the reaction immediately. These are the early signs of an insulin reaction:

- feeling hungry
- feeling sick-to-the-stomach
- a headache
- weakness
- shaking
- sweating
- double vision or blurred vision
- a change in mood or the way you act

The signs of an insulin reaction occur fast, usually within 10–15 minutes. When they happen you must eat or drink food *RIGHT AWAY*. You can take:

- ½ cup orange juice, or
- ½ cup of regular (soft drink or soda) pop, or
- 2 pieces of hard candy, or
- 6 Life Savers, or
- 5 sugar cubes, or
- 2 tablespoons of raisins, or
- 2 teaspoons of honey, or
- an over the counter insulin reaction product.

These are suggestions. You can use any food with quick-acting sugar in it.

This type of food will raise your blood sugar. You should feel better within five minutes. If you do not feel better, eat or drink the same amount again.

If the early signs of a reaction are not treated right away, they will become worse. You may begin to feel:

- confused
- unsteady on your feet
- drowsy
- unable to speak clearly

YOU MUST RAISE YOUR BLOOD SUGAR IMMEDIATELY!

Eat or drink any of the foods listed above if you feel a reaction coming on. If you are a family member or friend of a diabetic who has these symptoms, you may have to help treat the reaction. If the person cannot swallow or will not swallow, you should try to give the person corn syrup, honey (2 teaspoons), or a product called Glutose®. *Glutose* is a sweet, gel-like substance available in a squeeze bottle. You can buy glutose at your drugstore to have on hand in case of insulin reactions. If a diabetic passes out, *Glucagon*® may be given by someone else. Glucagon is injected into the body. You need a doctor's prescription to buy Glucagon. Ask your doctor or nurse when and how to use Glucagon.

Always treat the signs of a reaction immediately. If you do not, you may pass out. You can prevent most insulin reactions by following these rules:

- Eat the correct amounts and types of food.
- Eat your meals and snacks on time. If your meals are delayed for some reason, eat one or more exchanges now. If your evening meal is delayed, you may eat your bedtime snack at your usual mealtime.
- Eat one fruit exchange for each hour of exercise such as swimming, running, tennis, heavy housework, skiing, or other similar activity. (See Chapter Two on exercise.)

- Do not take extra insulin or pills unless your doctor tells you to.
- Do not skip meals or snacks.
- Always carry sugar or candy with you in case of a reaction.

Below are some facts about taking insulin or oral agents you should also know.

SAFE DRIVING

You want to avoid having an insulin reaction while driving. We suggest you *eat one fruit exchange for each two hours of driving*. If you have not eaten within two hours before you drive, eat something just before you leave.

We also suggest that if you take insulin you contact the Driver's License Division of the State Department of Public Safety. You may be asked to have your doctor send a letter to this department. Your doctor will state that you are under his or her care and that your diabetes is controlled by insulin. In case you are in an accident, this letter will protect you from unfair accusations. There is no reason you cannot drive if you keep your diabetes under control.

ALCOHOL

Ask your doctor if you can drink alcohol, and how much alcohol is safe for you. Remember that alcohol is high in calories and low in food value. Alcohol affects diabetes in a surprising way. When you have a drink your blood sugar will first go down, then it will slowly rise. These changes in your blood sugar could mean problems for you. When the blood sugar is too low you could have an insulin reaction. Some symptoms of an insulin reaction are not very different from symptoms of being drunk. People around you may not realize that you are having a reaction.

- To prevent an insulin reaction, always eat your meal with the drink, or eat a starch exchange with the drink.

TRAVEL

Changes in mealtimes, diets, and exercise often occur when traveling. You should always be prepared to treat an insulin reaction when away from home by carrying a form of sugar with you.

You can discuss the ethnic foods of the country you will visit with your dietitian. Also discuss any changes that might or will take place in your diabetes control with your doctor.

IDENTIFICATION

All diabetics should carry a form of identification which states, "I am a diabetic" in their wallet or purse. Many identification cards give instructions for treating an insulin reaction and phone numbers for your doctor or next of kin.

Diabetics who take pills or insulin should also wear a bracelet or neck chain with the Medic-Alert symbol. This symbol will alert medical personnel and other persons to the special needs of the diabetic in cases of accident, injury, or insulin reaction. Medical identification aids may be purchased in most jewelry stores.

Evaluate Yourself 1

1. What is an insulin reaction?

2. What are five symptoms of an insulin reaction?

3. What should you do if you have an insulin reaction?

4. When is a reaction most likely to happen?

5. How can you prevent an insulin reaction?

Answers to Evaluate Yourself 1

1. An insulin reaction is a condition where not enough sugar is in your blood, or there is a sudden drop in your blood sugar.
2. Early symptoms of an insulin reaction are feeling hungry, feeling sick-to-the-stomach, having a headache, weakness, shaking, sweating, double vision, or a mood change. Later symptoms are confusion, drowsiness, slurred speech, and staggering.
3. If you have a reaction, eat some food or drink some liquid containing sugar immediately.
4. A reaction is most likely to happen if you do not eat enough food, if you do not eat your meals or snacks on time, if you exercise without eating extra food, or if you take too much insulin or too many pills.
5. Most of the time, you can prevent a reaction by eating on time, following your meal plan, eating extra food when you exercise, and by taking the right amount of insulin or pills.

4

Ketoacidosis and Hyperosmolar Coma

KETOACIDOSIS

Diabetics often ask if they will go into a diabetic coma. If a person follows the guidelines of good control, coma should not occur. Diabetic coma is also called *diabetic acidosis or ketoacidosis.* We will use the term ketoacidosis. This term describes what occurs when diabetes goes out of control.

You may recall that when the cells of the body do not receive sugar for energy they begin to burn another source of energy: fat. When cells burn fat, *ketones* (poisons) are produced. When ketones and sugar build up in the body, they can lead to ketoacidosis. The following drawings will show you what happens in this process.

1. Food turns into sugar.

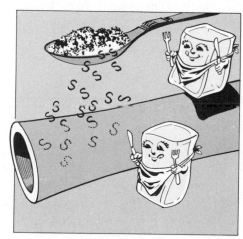

2. Sugar does not enter the cells because there is not enough insulin to open the cell door.

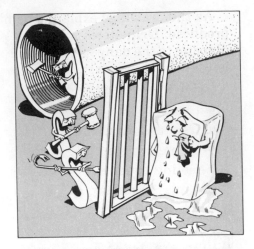

3. Blood sugar rises above normal; sugar spills into urine.

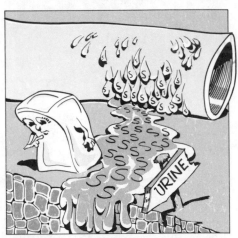

4. Cells burn fat and produce ketones. Ketones spill into blood and urine.

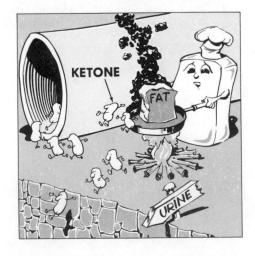

As the drawings explain, the blood sugar is high before ketones are produced. Urine tests will show ½%, 1%, or 2% results. This alerts the diabetic to the danger signals of high blood sugar and ketoacidosis. This is the time to contact your doctor, before the problem becomes worse.

Symptoms of *high blood sugar* are:

- thirst
- frequent urination
- blurred vision
- feeling tired
- pain, numbness, or tingling in fingers and/or toes
- sugar in the urine.

If these symptoms go untreated, signs of ketoacidosis may occur. These signs include:

- ketones and sugar in the urine
- flu symptoms (nausea, vomiting, stomach pain, diarrhea)
- hot, dry skin
- deep, rapid breathing
- fruity odor on the breath
- sleepy feeling, possibly leading to coma.

These symptoms can occur slowly, over days. If the danger signals are not heeded, ketoacidosis can lead to death.

A tool preventing ketoacidosis is urine or self blood sugar testing. Sugar and ketones in the urine are danger signals. These signals can mean high blood sugar and ketoacidosis. Let's recall our basic rules of urine testing:

1. Test your urine four times daily, before meals and bedtime.
2. Test freshly-made urine (second-voided specimen).
3. Record your results.
4. If urine sugar is ½%, 1% or 2%, or blood sugar is over 240mg. percent, test for ketones.
5. If urine sugar is ½%, 1%, or 2% or blood sugar is over 240mg. percent (with no ketones) for two days at every testing, call your doctor.
6. If urine sugar is ½%, 1%, or 2% *with ketones,* call your doctor within 24 hours.

Ketoacidosis may occur in any diabetic. It is most likely to occur when:
1. There is not enough insulin.
   - You measure the wrong amount of insulin.
   - You forget to take your insulin.
   - Your diabetes changes because of illness, weight gain, growth, or stress.

2. There is too much sugar.
   - You eat more food daily than your meal plan allows.
3. There is physical or emotional stress.
   - Flu, colds, or emotional upset may cause the blood sugar to rise.
   - Also, accidents, heart attacks, surgery, and pregnancy.
   - In times of stress you must be alert to symptoms of high blood sugar and ketoacidosis. You must still take your insulin or oral agent. You must still test your urine or blood.

Ketoacidosis is a serious health problem. It can be prevented. *Know* and *observe* the signs of *high blood sugar!*

HYPEROSMOLAR COMA

Hyperosmolar coma occurs most often in older adults with type II diabetes. It can also occur in older persons with undetected diabetes. Their blood sugar levels may reach very high levels. They do not develop ketoacidosis, so no ketones are present in the urine. For this reason hyperosmolar coma is sometimes called **nonketotic coma.** Most of the time, they do not take insulin. Their diabetes is controlled with oral pills and/or diet alone.

Hyperosmolar coma develops without the appearance of ketones in the urine. Do not wait for your urine test to test positive for ketones before you begin to worry about the bad effects that a very high blood sugar can have on your health. This problem is caused by some event that increases the body's need for insulin. This may be an acute infection, fever, fluid loss from diarrhea or vomiting, accident, stroke, or physical or emotional stress. It can also bbe caused by eating large amounts of sugar, taking large doses of steroids, diuretics, or tranquilizers and/or poor kidney function.

The word HYPEROSMOLAR means that the blood has become very concentrated. As the blood sugar rises to high levels, water is drawn from cells and tissues. The extra water is passed off in the urine with added sugar causing the early symptoms of extreme thirst or dehydration. This is a serious health problem that needs medical treatment right away. It can be a fatal complication of diabetes.

The symptoms of hyperosmolar coma are:

- urine high in sugar without ketones
- severe thirst
- dehydration
- dry mouth
- shallow breathing
- fatigue
- flushed, dry skin
- mental confusion and drowsiness
- unconsciousness

In order to treat hyperosmolar coma, a diabetic person requires hospital care without delay. During successful treatment, you will receive replacement of lost fluid and have your blood sugar controlled. Also, the treatment of the underlying illness will be started.

Prevention is much easier than treatment. Notify your doctor right away if the above symptoms occur. Family members of the older adult with diabetes should be alert to the symptoms of this type of coma. The diabetic person should not wait for urine ketones to appear before help is sought. Prompt treatment is extremely important. You can prevent hyperosmolar coma through careful, daily monitoring of your diabetes control.

STUDY QUESTIONS

Evaluate Yourself 1

1. What are five symptoms of high blood sugar?

2. What are five symptoms of ketoacidosis?

3. How can you prevent ketoacidosis?

4. What are five symptoms of hyperosmolar coma?

Answers to Evaluate Yourself 1

1. Symptoms of high blood sugar include:
   - thirst
   - frequent urination
   - blurred vision
   - feeling tired
   - pain, numbness, tingling in fingers and/or toes
   - sugar in the urine

2. Symptoms of ketoacidosis are:
   - ketones and sugar in the urine
   - flu symptoms (nausea, vomiting, stomach pains, diarrhea)
   - hot, dry skin
   - deep, rapid breathing
   - fruity odor on the breath
   - sleepy feeling, possibly leading to coma

3. You can prevent ketoacidosis by:
   - urine or self blood sugar testing

- knowing when to call the doctor
- following a meal plan
- taking the right amount of insulin
- taking insulin at the same time every day. Stress can make the blood sugar rise. Be alert for symptoms and signs of high blood sugar.

4. Symptoms of hyperosmolar coma are:
- urine high in sugar without ketones
- severe thirst
- dry mouth
- weakness or fatigue
- mental confusion and drowsiness

II

HEALTHY EATING

5

Food Groups

YOUR MEAL PLAN

The food that you eat is the most important, and often the hardest part of diabetic control. Your meal plan is your personal way of eating throughout the day. It is a way to keep your food intake about the same from day to day.

Your meal plan is individualized. It is planned only for you. When your dietitian or nutritionist designs your plan, it is centered around the way you eat. Your meal plan takes into account your food likes, dislikes, and ethnic and religious practices. Your social, work, and activity lifestyle also will be worked in. The medication you take may also affect your meal plan.

You may need to alter your eating habits. If you do, keep these guidelines in mind:

1. You should not eat foods that contain a lot of sugar. These foods are sugar, honey, jam, and molasses. Other foods that contain extra sugar are canned fruit in heavy sugar syrup, sweetened fruit drinks, pie, pastry, sweet rolls, rich desserts, and beverages that contain sugar. There are times when it is all right to eat some of these foods. When you are ill, you may need to drink pop, soda, or soft drinks. See Chapter 9 on illness. During special times of year, like a birthday or the holidays, you may eat a piece of cake or a piece of fudge. Be sure to count the food exchanges!

2. You should not undereat or overeat. Try to eat all of the foods in your meal plan each day.

3. You should eat three meals a day. Also, eat any snacks that are planned for you.

4. You should eat your meals at about the same time each day.

5. You should not omit meals.

6. Contact your dietitian if you have any questions or problems about your meal plan. You may find that as your lifestyle changes, you want to alter your meal plan.

MEAL PLANNING

The meal plan tells you the number of servings to eat from each food group. The meal plan tells you when to eat.

The kinds of food that make up your meal plan are taken from the six food groups. The six food groups are *milk, fruit, vegetable, bread-starch, meat,* and *fat.*

The six food groups include all the nutrients that your body needs to stay healthy. Foods are grouped together because foods within each group have similar nutrients. Each serving of a food in the same group has the same carbohydrate, protein, and fat content. Each serving of food in the same group has the same caloric content.

The foods in one group may be substituted for each other. Do *not* substitute a food from one group for a food from another group. You can substitute one-half cup of orange juice for a peach. But, you can *not* substitute one-half cup of orange juice for one slice of bread. Orange juice and peaches are in the same food group—fruit. Bread is in the bread-starch group.

Everyone's eating habits change over a period of time. You may not eat the same foods in the winter as you do in the summer. It is a good idea to discuss your meal plan with a dietitian every once in a while. For instance, your meal plan for breakfast may be as follows:

- 1 fruit exchange
- 1 meat exchange
- 2 bread-starch exchanges
- 1 fat exchange
- 1 milk exchange

Then you can eat this if you want to:

- ½ cup orange juice (fruit)
- 1 boiled egg (meat)
- 1 slice of toast and ½ cup oatmeal (bread-starch exchanges)
- 1 teaspoon margarine (fat)
- 1 cup milk (milk)

Perhaps the only time you would have one meat exchange would be at breakfast. One meat exchange is equal to one egg. It can be the egg we planned above.

At dinner, a common serving is three meat exchanges.

3 meat exchanges are

**3 ounces chicken
(a leg & thigh;
a breast & wing)**

or

**a 2 ounce beef patty
and
¼ cup cottage cheese**

FOOD EXCHANGES

The food exchange or groups provide the nutrients that your body needs for good health. As mentioned under meal planning, foods are grouped together by their carbohydrate, protein, fat, and calorie content. The food groups are milk, fruit, vegetable, bread-starch, meat, and fat.

You can eat one food instead of another food from the same food group. Do not replace a food from one group for a food from another group. Each group has a different number of calories and nutrient content. For instance, one slice of bread has the same nutrients and calories as one-half cup of potato. You can eat one-half cup of mashed potatoes instead of one slice of bread. Or, you can eat any other food from the bread-starch group.

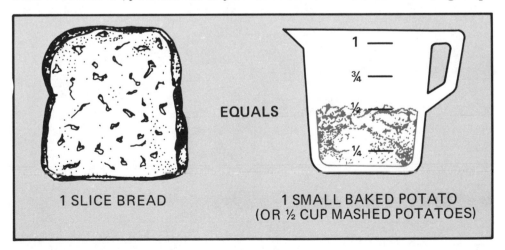

EQUALS

1 SLICE BREAD

1 SMALL BAKED POTATO
(OR ½ CUP MASHED POTATOES)

It is not correct to substitute a bread-starch serving for a meat serving. It is also not correct to substitute one bread-starch serving for a food in any other food group.

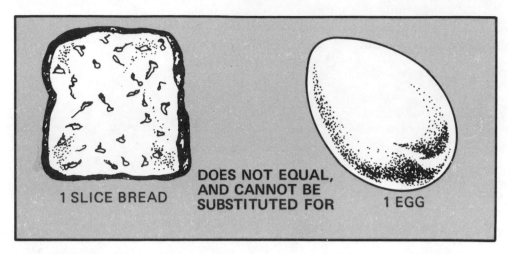

1 SLICE BREAD   DOES NOT EQUAL, AND CANNOT BE SUBSTITUTED FOR   1 EGG

You will receive a list of the six food groups from your dietitian (see below). Each food in a group may be called one food exchange or:

- one exchange,
- one unit,
- one serving,
- one substitute, or
- one portion.

Your meal plan will tell you if you may eat more than one exchange from a food group at your meals or snacks. For instance, if you have 2 bread-starch exchanges at your noon meal, you can eat:

- 1 slice of bread and ½ cup of peas,
- 1 cup of peas,
- or 2 slices of bread.

You can eat 2 servings of the same kind of food or you can eat one serving of each of two different foods.

YOUR PERSONAL MEAL PLAN

_____ calories a day

Snacks

Breakfast (_____)   **Morning (_____ AM)**
_____ meat exchange
_____ bread-starch exchange
_____ fruit exchange
_____ cups of milk

Lunch (_____)   **Afternoon (_____ PM)**
_____ meat exchange
_____ bread-starch exchange

_____ vegetable exchange
_____ fruit exchange
_____ cups of milk

Dinner (_____)   **Night** (_____ PM)
_____ meat exchange
_____ bread-starch exchange
_____ vegetable exchange
_____ fruit exchange
_____ cups of milk

Eat_____fat exchanges a day.

You can eat 20 extra calories at three different times during the day.

YOUR PERSONAL MENU PLANNING

Plan one day's menu for home on this page.

BREAKFAST

_____ fruit exchange
_____ meat exchange
_____ bread-starch exchange

_____ fat choice
_____ cups of _____ milk

LUNCH

_____ meat exchange
_____ bread-starch exchange

_____ vegetable exchange
_____ vegetable exchange
_____ fruit exchange
_____ fat exchange
_____ cups of _____ milk

DINNER

_____ meat exchange
_____ bread-starch exchange

_____ vegetable exchange
_____ vegetable exchange
_____ fruit exchange
_____ fat exchange
_____ cups of _____ milk

SNACKS

Morning   Afternoon   Evening

MILK EXCHANGE

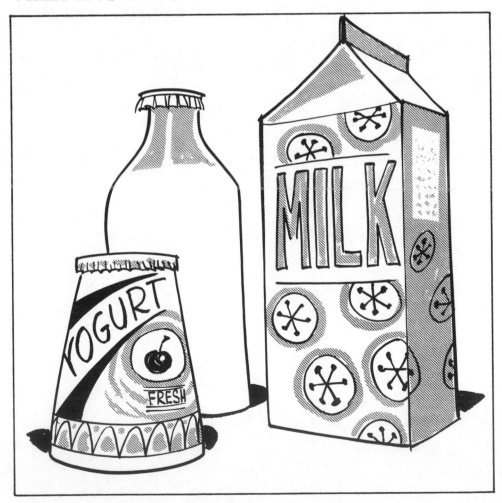

One cup or 8 ounces of milk contains 12 grams of carbohydrate and 8 grams of protein. Fat will vary with the kind of milk.

The calories will also vary because of the fat content:

- 1 cup of skim or non-fat milk has 80 calories
- 1 cup of low-fat or 2% milk has 125 calories
- 1 cup of whole milk has 170 calories

You can use milk in your meal plan to drink. You can add milk to cereal, coffee, tea, and other foods.

The list below shows the amount of milk to use for *one* serving. One serving is equal to 8 ounces.

- **Non-fat Fortified Milk**

skim or non-fat milk	1 cup
powdered (non-fat dry, before adding liquid)	⅓ cup
canned, evaporated—skim milk	½ cup
buttermilk made from skim milk	1 cup
yogurt made from skim milk (plain, unflavored)	1 cup

- **Low-fat Fortified Milk**

1% fat-fortified milk	1 cup
2% fat-fortified milk	1 cup
yogurt made from 2% fortified milk (plain, unflavored)	1 cup

- **Whole Milk**

whole milk	1 cup
canned, evaporated whole milk	½ cup
buttermilk made from whole milk	1 cup
yogurt made from whole milk (plain, unflavored)	1 cup

VEGETABLE EXCHANGE

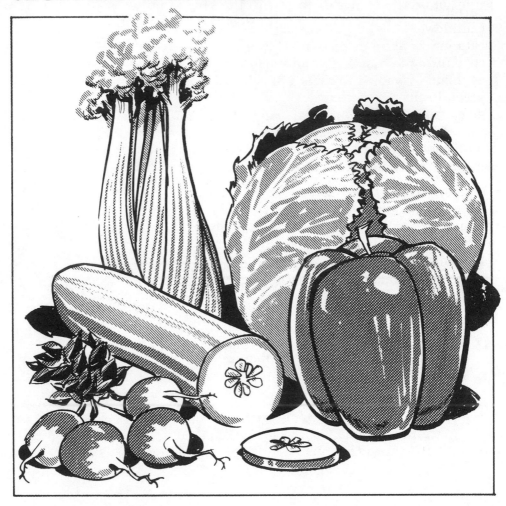

One serving of vegetables contains five grams of carbohydrate and two grams of protein and 28 calories.

Dark green and deep yellow vegetables are good sources of vitamin A. You should eat one serving of a food high in vitamin A every other day.

The group listed below shows you the kinds of vegetables to use for one serving.

One serving equals ½ cup cooked

asparagus	greens:	rutabaga
bean sprouts	beets	sauerkraut
beets	chard	string beans
broccoli	collards	summer squash
brussel sprouts	dandelion	tomatoes
cabbage	kale	tomato juice

Greens (cont.)

carrots	mustard	turnips
cauliflower	spinach	vegetable juice
celery	turnip	cocktail
cucumbers	mushrooms	yellow beans
eggplant	okra	zucchini
green beans	onions	
green peppers	rhubarb	

These raw vegetables may be used as desired if you take small servings

chicory	lettuce
Chinese cabbage	parsley
cucumber	radishes
endive	watercress
escarole	

Starchy vegetables are found in the bread-starch exchange group.

FRUIT EXCHANGE

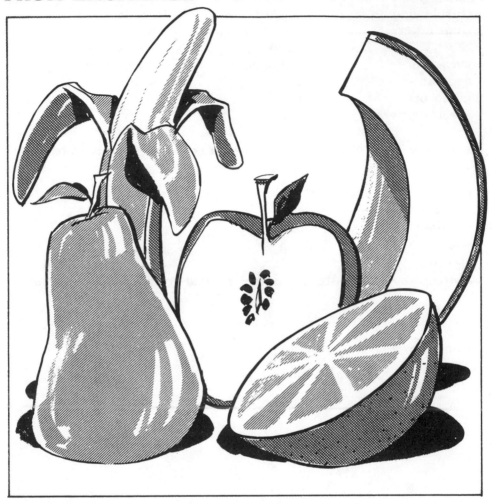

One serving of fruit contains 10 grams of carbohydrate and 40 calories. You can use fruits that are fresh, dried, canned, frozen, cooked, or raw. Do not use fruit that has sugar added to it. Citrus fruits and fruit juices contain vitamin C. You should eat one serving of fruit that has vitamin C in it every day.

The group below shows the kinds of fruits that you can use. Each amount listed is for *one serving*. The portions vary because the amount of natural sugar in fruit varies.

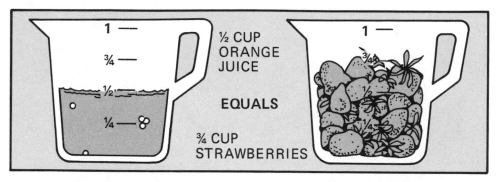

½ CUP
ORANGE
JUICE

EQUALS

¾ CUP
STRAWBERRIES

For example:

Orange juice has more sugar or carbohydrate than strawberries. Therefore, you must eat a smaller portion of orange juice to equal one fruit choice.

Other fruit exchanges are:

apple	1 small	grape juice	¼ cup
apple juice	⅓ cup	mango	½ small
applesauce		melons	
(unsweetened)	½ cup	canteloupe	¼ small
apricots, fresh	2 medium	honeydew	⅛ medium
apricots, dried	4 halves	watermelon	1 cup
banana	½ small	nectarine	1 small
berries		orange	1 small
blackberries	½ cup	orange juice	½ cup
blueberries	½ cup	papaya	¾ cup
raspberries	½ cup	peach	1 medium
strawberries	¾ cup	pear	1 small
cherries	10 large	persimmon, native	1 medium
cider	⅓ cup	pineapple	½ cup
dates	2	pineapple juice	⅓ cup
figs, fresh	1	plums	2 medium
figs, dried	1	prunes	2 medium
grapefruit	½	prune juice	¼ cup
grapefruit juice	½ cup	raisins	2 tbsp
grapes, large	12	tangerine	1 medium
grapes, small	24		

BREAD-STARCH EXCHANGE

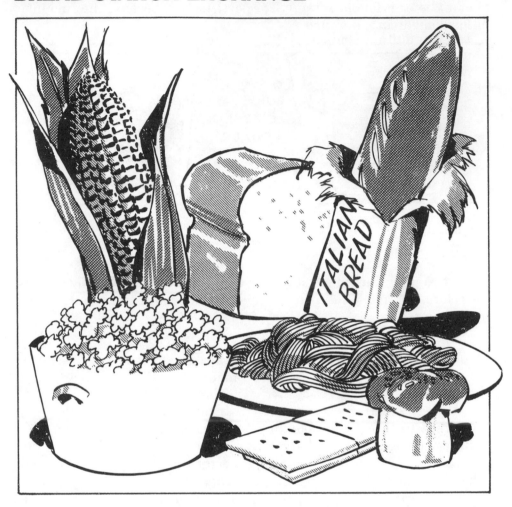

The bread-starch group includes breads, cereals, and starchy vegetables. One serving from the bread-starch group contains 15 grams of carbohydrate, 2 grams of protein, and 68 calories. Starchy vegetables are placed in this group because they contain the same amount of carbohydrate and protein as the other foods in this group.

The list of bread-starch foods here shows the kinds of breads, cereals, starchy vegetables, and prepared foods that you can eat. Each amount that is listed is *one serving*.

Breads

white, French, and Italian	1 slice
whole wheat	1 slice
rye or pumpernickel	1 slice
raisin	1 slice

Dried Beans, Peas, and Lentils

beans, peas, lentils (cooked and dried)	½ cup
baked beans, no pork (canned)	¼ cup

Breads (cont.)

bagel, small	½
English muffin, small	½
plain roll, bread	1
frankfurter roll	½
hamburger bun	½
dried bread crumbs	3 tbsp
tortilla, 6 inch	1

Cereal

grapenuts	¼ cup
bran flakes	½ cup
other ready-to-eat unsweetened cereal	¾ cup
puffed cereal (unfrosted)	1 cup
cereal (cooked)	½ cup
grits (cooked)	½ cup
rice or barley (cooked)	½ cup
pasta (cooked) spaghetti, noodles, macaroni	½ cup
popcorn (popped, no fat added)	
small kernel	1½ cups
large kernel	3 cups
cornmeal (dry)	2 tbsp
flour	2½ tbsp
wheat germ	¼ cup

Crackers

arrowroot	3
graham, 2½" square	2
matzoth, 4x6"	½
oyster	20
pretzels, 3⅛" long x ⅛" diameter	25
rye wafers, 2"x3½"	3
saltines	6
soda, 2½" square	4

Starchy Vegetables

corn	⅓ cup
corn on cob (3–4")	1 small
lima beans	½ cup
parsnips	⅔ cup
peas, green (canned or frozen)	½ cup
potato, white	1 small
potato, mashed	½ cup
pumpkin	¾ cup
winter squash, acorn or butternut	½ cup
yam or sweet potato	¼ cup

Prepared Foods

biscuit 2" diameter (omit 1 fat exchange)	1
corn bread, 2"x2"x1" (omit 1 fat exchange)	1
corn muffin, 2" diameter (omit 1 fat exchange)	1
crackers, round butter type (omit 1 fat exchange)	5
muffin, plain small (omit 1 fat exchange)	1
Chinese noodles (omit 1 fat exchange)	½ cup
potatoes, french fried 2 to 3½" long (omit 1 fat exchange)	8
potato or corn chips (omit 2 fat exchanges)	15
pancake, 5" x ½" (omit 1 fat exchange)	1
waffle, 5" x ½" (omit 1 fat exchange)	1

MEAT EXCHANGE

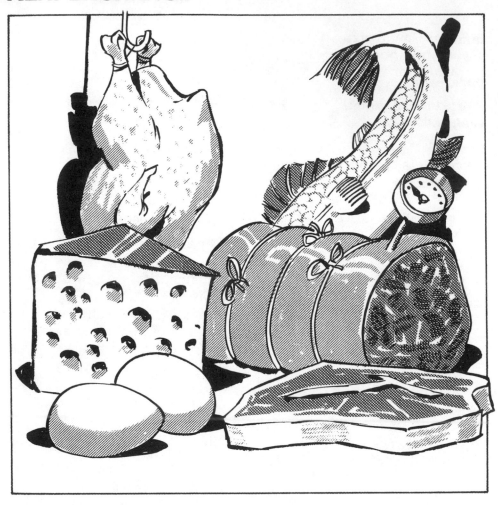

The meat group includes lean (low-fat) meat, medium-fat meat, and high-fat meat. It is better to choose most of your meats and meat exchanges from the lean and medium-fat groups.

Each group listed below shows the amount of meat and meat exchange you can use for one serving. Each group lists the kind of meat and meat choices that are lean meat, medium-fat meat, or high-fat meat choices.

Lean Meat

One serving, or one ounce, contains 7 grams of protein, 3 grams of fat, and 55 calories.

beef:	baby beef (very lean), chipped beef, chuck, flank steak, tenderloin, plate ribs,	1 oz

	plate skirt steak, round, all rump cuts, spare ribs, tripe	
lamb:	leg, rib, sirloin, roast and chops, shank, shoulder	1 oz
pork:	leg (such as whole rump or center shank), center slices of smoked ham	1 oz
veal:	leg, loin, rib, shank, shoulder, cutlets	1 oz
poultry:	chicken, turkey, Cornish hen, guinea hen, pheasant without the skin	1 oz
fish:	any fresh or frozen	1 oz
	canned salmon, tuna, mackerel, crab and lobster	¼ cup
	clams, oysters, scallops, shrimp	5 or 1 oz
	sardines, drained	3
cheese:	cheese that contains less than 5% butterfat like Sap Sago, Gammelost, Countdown cheese	1 oz
	cottage cheese, dry and 2% butterfat	¼ cup
	dried beans and peas (omit 1 bread exchange)	½ cup

Medium-fat Meat

One serving or one ounce of medium-fat meat contains 7 grams of protein, 5 grams of fat, and 73 calories.

beef:	ground (15% fat), corned beef (canned), rib eye, round (ground commercial)	1 oz
pork:	loin (all cuts tenderloin), shoulder arm (picnic), shoulder blade, Boston butt, Canadian bacon, boiled ham	1 oz

liver, heart, kidney, and sweetbreads (these are high in cholesterol) — 1 oz

cottage cheese, creamed — ¼ cup

Cheese:	Mozzarella, Ricotta, farmer's cheese, Neufchatel	1 oz
	Parmesan	1 oz
		3 tbsp
	cottage cheese, creamed	¼ cup

egg (high in cholesterol) — 1

peanut butter (omit 2 fat exchanges) — 2 tbsp

High-fat Meat

One serving or one ounce of high-fat meat contains 7 grams of protein, 7 grams of fat, and 91 calories.

beef:	brisket, corned beef (brisket), ground beef (more than 20% fat), chuck (ground commercial), roasts (rib), steaks (club and rib)	1 oz
lamb:	breast	1 oz
pork:	spare ribs, loin (back ribs) pork (ground), country style ham, deviled ham	1 oz
veal:	breast	1 oz
poultry:	capon, duck, goose	1 oz
cheese:	cheddar types	1 oz
cold cuts		4½″ x ⅛″ slice
frankfurter		1 small

FAT EXCHANGE

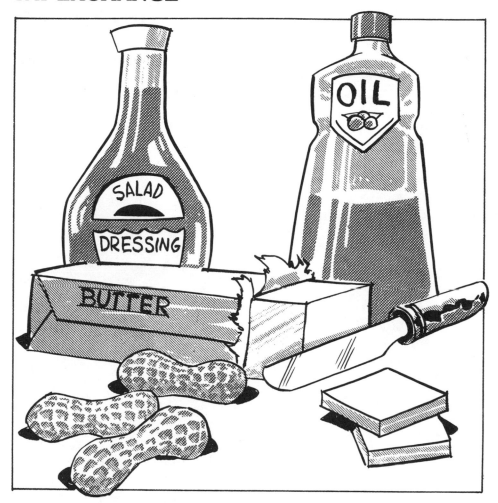

One serving of fat contains 5 grams of fat and 45 calories.

There are two fat groups. The first group lists those foods that are high in *polyunsaturated* and *unsaturated fat*. The second group lists those foods that are high in saturated fat. The two groups show the kinds and amounts of food to use for *one serving*.

Polyunsaturated Fat

margarine, soft, tub, or stick	1 tsp	mayonnaise	1 tsp
avocado (4″ dia.)	⅛	olives	5 small
oil, corn, cottonseed, safflower, soy, or sunflower	1 tsp	almonds	10 whole
		pecans	2 large whole
oil, olive	1 tsp	peanuts	
oil, peanut	1 tsp	Spanish	20 whole
		Virginia	10 whole

French dressing	1 tbsp	walnuts	6 small
Italian dressing	1 tbsp	nuts, other	6 small

Saturated Fat

margarine, regular stick	1 tsp	low cal dressing	2 tbsp
butter	1 tsp	creamy dressing	½ tbsp
bacon fat	1 tsp	lard	1 tsp
bacon, crisp	1 strip	salad dressing,	
cream, light	2 tbsp	mayonnaise type	2 tsp
non-dairy cream		salt pork	¾" cube
substitute	2 tbsp		
cream, sour	2 tbsp		
gravy	2 tbsp		
cream cheese	1 tbsp		

NUTRIENTS IN GRAMS

For One Serving

food exchange	carbo-hydrate	pro-tein	fat	calories
milk non-fat	12	8		80
vegetable	5	2		28
fruit	10			40
bread-starch	15	2		68
meat, lean		7	3	55
meat, medium-fat		7	5	73
meat, high-fat		7	7	91
fat			5	45

DIETARY FIBER

Dietary fiber is that portion of food that you do not digest. It is not absorbed into the bloodstream. Fiber gives plants their shape. Fiber forms the outer coat to protect the plant.

Research suggests that a High Carbohydrate, High Fiber (HCF) diet helps control your blood sugar levels. A high fiber diet can also decrease insulin needs. The way your diabetes is controlled can change if you are on a high fiber diet. Discuss the benefits of a high fiber diet with your doctor and discuss your meal plan with your dietitian.

Usually, foods that are not refined contain more fiber than foods that are highly refined. Some fiber is removed when a food is processed. For instance, whole wheat bread contains more fiber than white bread because white bread is processed more than whole wheat bread.

A good source of fiber is raw fruit that still has the skin, like an apple. The skin of other fruits, such as grapes, adds fiber to your diet. And the seeds in a fruit, like strawberries, also adds fiber. Raw and cooked vegetables, such as corn and beans, are high in fiber. If you eat the stems and leaves, you will also add extra fiber to your diet, such as lettuce and brussel sprouts. If you adhere to a high fiber meal plan, you will consume less fat and cholesterol, and three times the fiber of the normal American diet. The greatest effect on your diabetes control seems to be achieved when you consume about 70 percent of your total calories as carbohydrate. It is a good idea to closely monitor your urine or blood glucose levels. You may need to reduce your insulin or pill dose.

HIGH FIBER MEAL PLAN

The food groups that contain fiber are the bread–starch group, the fruit group, and the vegetable group. The milk group, the meat group (meat and meat substitutes) and the fat group do not add any fiber to your diet. The milk group is the only food group that contains carbohydrate that does not contain fiber. Your dietitian or nutritionist will take these guidelines into account in order to design your high fiber meal plan.

Guidelines to follow for a high fiber meal plan are:

- Increase your total carbohydrate intake to 55–60 percent of your total calories.
- Eat 40 grams of plant fiber a day. Eat 20–25 grams of plant fiber a day for each 1,000 calories (40–50 grams for 2,000 calories).
- Consume about 18–23 percent of your total calories as protein.
- Decrease protein foods (meat and meat substitutes) to about 4–6 ounces per day. If fish is chosen, you can eat about 8 ounces a day.
- Decrease your fat intake to 20–30 percent of your total calories.
- Decrease or omit the fat you add to your food. Try to avoid invisible fat, like marbled meat, whole milk, and most cheese.

The High Carbohydrate, High Fiber (HCF) exchange list here contains nine food groups. There are more food groups in order to better determine the fiber content of your diet. Foods that contain about the same amount of fiber are grouped together. The bread–starch group is divided into breads, cereals, starchy vegetables, and beans.

You use the high fiber exchange list in the same manner as the other exchange list. (See Your Meal Plan and Meal Planning).

Here are the nine food groups and the fiber, carbohydrate, protein, fat, and caloric content per serving.

Milk

skim (non-fat) milk, buttermilk, evaporated skim milk, plain low-fat or skim milk yogurt

One exchange (1 cup) contains:
0 grams FIBER
12 grams carbohydrate
8 grams protein
0 grams fat
80 calories

Vegetables

May be fresh, frozen, or canned. Do not add extra fat, sauces, glazes, cheese, or other foods. This list shows the kinds of vegetables to use for *one exchange or serving*.

One exchange contains:
2 grams FIBER
5 grams carbohydrate
2 grams protein
0 grams fat
28 calories

One serving is ½ to ¾ cup cooked or 1–2 cups raw

asparagus	greens:	rutabaga
bean sprouts	beets	sauerkraut
beets	chard	string beans
broccoli	collards	summer squash
brussel sprouts	dandelion	tomatoes
cabbage	kale	tomato juice
carrots	mustard	turnips
cauliflower	spinach	vegetable juice
celery	turnip	cocktail
cucumbers	mushrooms	yellow beans
eggplant	okra	zucchini
green beans	onions	
green peppers	rhubarb	

RAW VEGETABLES

chicory	lettuce
Chinese cabbage	parsley
endive	radishes
escarole	watercress

Starchy vegetables are found in the bread–starch exchange group.

Fruits

One fruit exchange contains:

2 grams FIBER
10 grams carbohydrate
0 grams protein or fat
40 calories

Use raw or canned fruits in their own juice, unsweetened or artificially sweetened. Fruit juices with pulp and canned fruit contain less fiber than raw fruit. One fruit serving is:

apple	1 small	grape juice	¼ cup
apple juice	⅓ cup	mango	½ small
applesauce		melons	
(unsweetened)	½ cup	canteloupe	¼ small
apricots, fresh	2 medium	honeydew	⅛ medium
apricots, dried	4 halves	watermelon	1 cup
banana	½ small	nectarine	1 small
berries		orange	1 small
blackberries	½ cup	orange juice	½ cup
blueberries	½ cup	papaya	¾ cup
raspberries	½ cup	peach	1 medium
strawberries	¾ cup	pear	1 small
cherries	10 large	persimmon, native	1 medium
cider	⅓ cup	pineapple	½ cup
dates	2	pineapple juice	⅓ cup
figs, fresh	1	plums	2 medium
figs, dried	1	prunes	2 medium
grapefruit	½	prune juice	¼ cup
grapefruit juice	½ cup	raisins	2 tbsp
grapes, large	12	tangerine	1 medium
grapes, small	24		

Breads and Grains

Use whole grain breads and crackers; whole meal flour, such as the stone ground variety, or whole wheat flour; whole meal, whole wheat, or rye bread; rye crackers; and bran muffins.

BREAD

rye or whole wheat bread	1 slice
graham crackers	2 squares
rye crackers (Rye Krisp)	3 squares
muffins, bran, oat, corn	½ muffin
popcorn	3 cups
pumpernickel bread	1 slice
whole meal bread	1 slice
whole wheat crackers	6
whole wheat rolls	1
wheat bran	½ cup

(12 grams fiber instead of 2 grams)

One exchange contains:
2 grams FIBER
15 grams carbohydrate
2 grams protein
1 gram fat
77 calories

CEREALS

Excellent sources of fiber are:

rolled whole oats, cooked (oatmeal)	½ cup
Ralstons or rolled whole wheat, cooked	½ cup
wheat flakes (Wheaties)	¾ cup
Shredded Wheat	1 biscuit
Puffed Wheat	1¼ cup
Bran Flakes (40% bran)	¾ cup
Post Toasties	1 cup
Grapenut Flakes	⅔ cup
Bran Flakes with Raisins	⅓ cup
Grapenuts	¼ cup
Corn Flakes	¾ cup
Corn Bran	½ cup
grits	¼ cup
Bran Chex	⅓ cup
Corn Chex	¾ cup
Total	¾ cup
All Bran or 100% Bran*	⅓ cup
Bran Buds*	½ cup

(*8 grams fiber instead of 3 grams)

One exchange contains:
3 grams FIBER
15 grams carbohydrate
2 grams protein
1 gram fat
77 calories

STARCHY VEGETABLES

corn, cooked	½ cup

Starchy Vegetables (cont.)

parsnips, cooked	¾ cup
sweet potatoes, cooked	¼ cup
potatoes, white, cooked	1 small
brown rice, cooked	⅓ cup
barley, cooked	½ cup
squash, winter	½ cup
peas	½ cup
cracked wheat (Bulgur)	¼ cup

One exchange contains:
3 grams FIBER
15 grams carbohydrate
2 grams protein
1 gram fat
77 calories

Beans

Beans are an excellent source of protein, carbohydrate, minerals, and fiber.

kidney beans, cooked	½ cup
lima beans, cooked	½ cup
white beans, cooked	½ cup
lentils, cooked	½ cup
pinto beans, cooked	½ cup
navy beans, cooked	½ cup

One exchange contains:
8 grams FIBER
15 grams carbohydrate
6 grams protein
1 gram fat
93 calories

1 bean exchange = 1 bread exchange
2 bean exchanges = 2 breads + 1 lean meat exchange

Meat

One exchange contains:
0 grams FIBER
9 grams protein
2 grams fat
0 grams carbohydrate
54 calories

lean beef, trimmed (tenderloin, rump, round, flank)	1 ounce
pork, lean ham or lean roast or chops	1 ounce
poultry, chicken or turkey	1 ounce
low-fat cottage cheese or skim milk cheeses	½ cup or 1 ounce
tuna, water-packed	¼ cup
egg whites (2 equal 1 egg)	one
fish, such as cod, flounder, trout	1 ounce
ground chuck or ground round	1 ounce

Trim meat well before cooking. Bake, broil, stew or boil. Do not fry.

Nuts and seeds like pumpkin, sesame, and/or sunflower seeds contain fiber.

nuts	1 oz (¼ cup)
seeds	1 oz (¼ cup)

One exchange of nuts and seeds contains:
3 grams FIBER
9 grams protein
16 grams fat
180 calories

Fat

One exchange contains:
0 grams FIBER
5 grams fat
0 grams carbohydrate and protein
45 calories

Polyunsaturated fats are margarines and oils made from corn, safflower, soybean oil, and liquid or soft tub margarines.

POLYUNSATURATED FAT		SATURATED FAT	
margarine, soft, tub or stick	1 tsp	margarine, regular stick	1 tsp
avocado (4″ dia.)	⅛	butter	1 tsp
oil, corn, cottonseed, safflower, soy, sunflower	1 tsp	bacon fat	1 tsp
		bacon, crisp	1 strip
oil, olive	1 tsp	cream, light	2 tbsp
oil, peanut	1 tsp	non-dairy cream substitute	2 tbsp
French dressing	1 tbsp	cream, sour	2 tbsp
Italian dressing	1 tbsp	gravy	2 tbsp
mayonnaise	1 tsp	cream cheese	1 tbsp
olives	5 small	low cal dressing	2 tbsp
		creamy dressing	½ tbsp
		lard	1 tsp
		salad dressing, mayonnaise type	2 tsp
		salt pork	¾″ cube

HIGH FIBER MEAL PLAN

Here is a sample 2000 calorie High Fiber meal plan.

Meal	Meal Plan	Menu	Grams of Fiber
Breakfast	1 cup skim milk	1 cup skim milk	0
	1 fruit exchange	1 orange	2
	2 cereal exchanges	1½ cup Total	6

	1 meat exchange	2 egg whites	0
	1 fat exchange	1 tsp margarine	0
Snack	1 fruit exchange	1 apple	2
Lunch	½ cup skim milk	½ cup skim milk	0
	1 fruit exchange	½ banana	2
	2 vegetable exchanges	½ cup green beans	2
		1 cup salad	2
	1 starchy vegetable exchange	½ cup peas	3
	2 bread exchanges	sandwich:	4
		2 slices bread, whole wheat	0
	2 meat exchanges	2 ounces chicken	
	2 fat exchanges	1 tsp margarine	0
		1 tbsp French dressing	
Snack	1 fruit exchange	½ cup orange juice	1
	1 bread exchange	3 cups popcorn	2
Dinner	1 fruit exchange	2 tbsp raisins	2
	2 vegetable exchanges	½ cup asparagus	2
		1 cup salad	2
	1 bread exchange	1 slice whole wheat bread	2
			2
	2 starchy vegetable exchanges	½ cup sweet potato	6
	1 bean exchange	½ cup pinto beans	8
	3 meat exchanges	3 ounces lean hamburger	0
	2 fat exchanges	2 tsp margarine	0
Snack	½ cup skim milk	½ cup skim milk	0
	1 fruit exchange	2 tbsp raisins	2
	2 bread exchanges	1 bran muffin	4

TOTAL: 56 grams of fiber

YOUR HIGH FIBER MEAL PLAN

_____ calories a day

Breakfast (_____)
_____ meat exchange
_____ bread exchange
_____ cereal exchange
_____ fruit exchange
_____ cups of milk

Snacks
Morning (_____AM)

Lunch (_____)

_____ meat exchange
_____ bean exchange
_____ bread exchange
_____ starchy vegetable
_____ vegetable exchange
_____ fruit exchange
_____ cups of milk

Afternoon (_____PM)

Dinner (_____)

_____ meat exchange
_____ bean exchange
_____ bread exchange
_____ starchy vegetable
_____ vegetable exchange
_____ fruit exchange
_____ cups of milk

Night (_____PM)

Eat_____fat exchanges a day.

You can eat 20 extra calories at 3 different times during the day.

HIGH FIBER MENU PLANNING

Plan one day's menu for home on this page.

BREAKFAST

_____ fruit exchange
_____ meat exchange
_____ bread exchange

_____ fat exchange
_____ cups milk (skim, 2%, whole)

LUNCH

_____ meat exchange
_____ bean exchange
_____ bread exchange

_____ starchy vegetable exchange

_____ vegetable exchange

_____ fruit exchange
_____ fat exchange
_____ cups milk (skim, 2%, whole)

DINNER

_____ meat exchange
_____ bean exchange
_____ bread exchange

_____ starchy vegetable exchange

_____ vegetable exchange

_____ fruit exchange
_____ fat exchange
_____ cups milk (skim, 2%, whole)

SNACKS

Morning
_____ fruit exchange
_____ bread exchange

_____ cups milk (skim, 2%, whole)

Afternoon
_____ fruit exchange
_____ bread exchange

_____ cups milk (skim, 2%, whole)

Evening
_____ fruit exchange
_____ bread exchange

_____ cups milk (skim, 2%, whole)

Evaluate Yourself 1

1. What are the general rules for control of your diet?

2. What would you do if a meal is delayed?

3. What would happen to your blood sugar if you skipped a meal?

4. What would happen to your blood sugar if you overate? If you underate?

5. What is an exchange?

6. Can you eat one slice of bread instead of ½ cup peaches?

7. What are the names of the food groups?

8. What food groups have the greatest effect on your blood sugar?

9. What food group contains the most calories?

10. Name six foods in the bread-starch food group.

11. Which of these foods are in the protein group: bacon or peanut butter?

12. What are the benefits of a high fiber eating plan?

13. Name the food groups that contain fiber.

14. What are the new food groups in the high fiber diet?

Answers to Evaluate Yourself 1

1. Eat the same amount of food at the same time.
   Do not overeat or undereat.
   Do not eat sugar.
   Do not skip meals.

2. Eat a food with carbohydrate or protein in it.
   Eat fruit, bread-starch food, milk, or meat.

3. Your blood sugar will fall and you may have an insulin reaction (see Chapter 3).

4. Overeat: your blood sugar will go too high.
   Undereat: your blood sugar will fall and you may have an insulin reaction (see Chapter 3).

5. One serving of food within each food group.

6. No. Bread is not in the fruit group.

7. Milk, Fruit, Vegetable, Bread-Starch, Meat, Fat.

8. The foods that contain carbohydrate: milk, fruit, vegetable, bread-starch.

9. Fat group.

10. See your bread-starch food group.

11. Peanut butter. It also contains a lot of fat. Bacon is in the fat group.

12. Decrease blood sugar and insulin dose.

13. Bread-starch, fruit, and vegetable food groups.

14. Bread, cereal, starchy vegetables, and beans.

6
Satisfying Your Sweet Tooth

SUGAR

You should avoid foods that contain only sugar. Sugar is a sweetened carbohydrate. Sugar does not contain any other nutrients, like vitamins or minerals. For example, orange juice contains fructose, which is a sugar. But it is a good food to drink because it also contains vitamin C.

Do *not* eat the foods listed below.

sugar	sorghum	regular gum
brown sugar	jam	marshmallows
corn sugar	jelly	cake frosting
corn sweetener	marmalade	filled cookies
honey	preserves	sweet rolls
molasses	regular soft drink	pastry
maple syrup	punch	filled or frosted dough-
corn syrup	fruit drinks	nuts
flavored syrups	candy	sugared cereal

You will see the following words on many food labels. They are chemical words for sugar. Each sugar contains 4 calories per gram.

maltose	lactose	sorbitol
glucose	levulose	mannitol
sucrose	dextrin	xylitol
dextrose	malto dextrins	invert sugar

Fructose

Fructose is the sugar that is found in fresh fruit, vegetables, and honey.

Fructose contains 4 calories per gram which is the same number of calories per gram found in sucrose. Refined fructose is limited in vitamin, mineral, and fiber content. But fruit which contains fructose does contain these nutrients.

Fructose is 15–80 percent sweeter than sucrose. The sweetness of fructose depends on its physical state and its temperature. For instance, fructose is sweeter when it is cold.

Beware of the use of the word fructose. Many food products are sweetened with high fructose corn sweetener which is not pure fructose. High fructose corn sweeteners can contain as much as 58 percent glucose. Be cautious when you read labels.

A diabetic person who is not overweight, and who is in good control, can eat moderate amounts of fructose in its pure form or when found in processed foods. Like any other food, the calories in fructose must be counted as part of the day's total. Consult with your physician or dietitian before you use fructose as a sweetening agent.

Sugar Substitutes

Saccharin

Saccharin, a non-nutritive sweetener, does not contain any calories. Some research has shown that it can cause cancer in animals.

It is a good idea to limit the amount of saccharin that you use. You can add it to your food or you can buy it in processed foods. There are many brand names of saccharin. Ask your dietitian for any information.

If you are an adult, try not to use more than one gram a day. The maximum amount is about the amount in 7 or 8 twelve-ounce cans of soft drink. If you are a child, try not to use more than one-half gram a day. This is the amount in about 3 or 4 twelve-ounce cans of soft drink.

Aspartame

Aspartame is the generic name of a low calorie sweetener made from protein. Aspartame is made from two amino acids, aspartic acid and phenylalanine. Aspartame is 180–200 times sweeter than sucrose. It provides the sweetness of one teaspoon of sugar with only $\frac{1}{10}$ of the calories. Therefore, this sweetener provides a minute number of calories to your diet.

Aspartame is not used in soft drinks. It is used in breakfast cereals, chewing gum, and powdered beverages. It is also found in whipped toppings, puddings, and gelatin. You can also use Aspartame to sweeten your own food.

LOOKING AT LABELS

Sugar is everywhere. No wonder you can get confused when you go shopping. And add to this, every supermarket has a diet shelf. This shelf is filled with more and more products that you can use in place of some other can or box. You may ask yourself, "What is safe to buy?"

Here are some things to remember when buying food:

- Read the entire label. Know the words meaning sugar by looking at your sugar list. Notice in what order the ingredients are listed. Look at the number of calories in a serving. Read the serving size and the protein, carbohydrate, and fat content. Shortening and coconut butter will give you lots of fat calories.
- Ingredients are listed from the largest amount to the smallest amount. You may find sugar or words meaning sugar in the list of ingredients. Sugar could be listed first on a label. This means the product has more sugar in it than any other ingredient. Cereals with a coating contain a lot of sugar.

Sugar could be farther down the label's ingredient list. This means the food contains a smaller amount of sugar. For instance, cornflakes contain sugar. The sugar in cornflakes is part of the total carbohydrate value of one bread-starch serving.

You can eat products that contain sugar. Also, you can eat products that contain sugar listed by other names. The sugar should be an ingredient farther down a label's list. Look for the food in your food groups or in your list of free foods.

dietetic does *not* mean diabetic

Dietetic does not mean that you can use the product as a free food. The product may have less sugar. It may also have less calories, less salt, and may have less fat or cholesterol.

If a product declares that it can be used in a diabetic diet, it must have this nutrition information statement on the label:

"Diabetics: This product may be useful in your diet on the advice of a physician."

Dietetic means that one or more ingredients usually found in a food have been changed or replaced. Dietetic can only be used if the product is also labeled as "low calorie." Here are some words you may find on a product:

Low calorie or low in calories. These statements mean that a common serving of a product has less than 40 calories per serving. A half slice of bread has less than 70 calories, but is not a common serving. Celery cannot be labeled low in calories. Nature made celery low in calories.

Low calorie or reduced calorie means that a product has at least one-third fewer calories than the product it is being compared to. This product must contain the same nutrients. The label must state the exact calorie difference between the reduced calorie product and the original product.

The terms below are often found on product labels:

Sugar-free means that a product does not contain table sugar. The product may have other kinds of sugars. Sorbitol or mannitol are sugars. Sorbitol and mannitol have calories. They will raise the blood sugar slower. There are products with sugar in them that you can eat.

The terms below are often found on product labels:

- **Sugar-free** can only be used if the product is also labeled "low calorie."
- **Sugarless** means that table sugar has not been used to make the product. Sugarless can only be used if the product is also labeled as "low calorie."
- **Artificially sweetened** means a product has been sweetened with a sugar substitute. Artificially sweetened can only be used if the product is also labeled "low calorie."
- **No sugar added** means that extra sugar has not been added to a product.
- **Unsweetened** means that extra sugar has not been added to a product.
- **Juice packed** means that a product is packed in a natural fruit juice.
- **Water packed** means that a product is packed in water. For example, let's talk about canned fruit. You can buy canned fruit in a variety of ways; artificially sweetened, packed in water, packed in syrup, and fruit packed in its' own juice.

Artificially sweetened canned fruit means that the fruit has been sweetened with a sugar substitute. When the fruit has been packed in water, water has been used in place of the syrup. If the fruit is packed in syrup, it has sugar added to it. If the fruit is packed in its own juice, any fruit juice has been used in place of the syrup.

Water packed and artificially sweetened fruit have the least number of calories in it. Juice packed fruit has more calories. If you use ⅓ to ½ cup of juice with your serving, you are eating one more fruit serving. Syrup packed fruit has the most calories: it has almost twice as many calories as those in water packed fruit.

FREE FOODS

Free foods are foods that:

- are very low in carbohydrate, protein, fat, and calories,
- are changed into only a small amount of blood sugar, and
- are labeled "dietetic" and have less than 20 calories a serving.

You can eat free foods at meal time to increase your number of food choices. You can also eat free foods between meals as snacks. Also, you do *not* have to eat free foods.

We can divide free foods into three groups:

- In the *first group* are foods that you can eat small amounts of any time you want.
- In the *second group* are foods that are free if you only eat a certain amount of them.
- In the *third group* are dietetic foods.

Free Foods—Group 1

These foods are very low in carbohydrate, protein, fat, and calories. These foods can add variety and flavor to your diet.

lettuce
celery
tomatoes
green pepper

herbs
spices
flavoring extracts
anagosta bitters
artificial sweetener
mustard, dry or prepared
poppyseed
sesame seed
meat tenderizers

coffee
tea
Sanka
diet pop, soft drink, or soda
club soda
artificially sweetened Kool-Aid
artificially sweetened lemonade

unsweetened gelatin
broth
unsweetened or dill pickles
unsweetened cranberries
unsweetened rhubarb
sugarless gum
meat sauces without sugar
vinegar
lemon
lemon juice
lime
lime juice
horseradish
tabasco sauce

Free Foods—Group 2

These foods all contain 20 calories.

low calorie salad dressing, 1 tablespoon
catsup, 1 tablespoon
barbecue sauce, 1 tablespoon
soy sauce, 1 tablespoon
taco sauce, 1 tablespoon
worcestershire sauce, 1 tablespoon
waffle type ice cream cone, 1 small
pretzels, "Veri-thin", 15
Cool-whip, 1 tablespoon
Bacos, 1 teaspoon
yogurt, plain, 2 tablespoons
cocoa powder, unsweetened, 2 teaspoons

Free Foods—Group 3

When you eat dietetic foods, *read the label*. Each brand name product will have a different number of calories in one serving. A dietetic food is a free food, if it has 20 calories or less in a serving. These foods include:

dietetic hard candies
dietetic jam, jelly, and preserves
dietetic syrup
low calorie whipped toppings

DESSERTS

When you eat desserts, you are eating extra sugar, fat, and calories. The extra sugar will raise your blood sugar more than usual. The extra calories will be more than your body needs that day.

It is all right for you to eat desserts once in a while. For special occasions you can eat a dessert three times a week. Do not eat all three dessert servings in one day. Keep in mind that you can eat your dessert in place of other foods in your meal plan.

Here is a list of the desserts that you can eat with the amount that you can eat, and the kind of food that you are eating.

Food	The number of exchanges from a food group
Cookies	
5 vanilla wafers	1 bread-starch exchange
5 ginger snaps	1 bread-starch exchange
4 arrowroots	1 bread-starch exchange
3 lorna doones	1 bread-starch exchange
3 two-inch peanut butter, chocolate chip, or oatmeal cookies	1 bread-starch exchange and 1 fat exchange
Cakes	
$\frac{1}{20}$ angel cake	1 bread-starch exchange
$\frac{5}{8}$ inch slice pound cake	1 bread-starch exchange and 1 fat exchange
2 inch square white or yellow cake	1 bread-starch exchange and 1 fat exchange
Plain cake doughnut, small	1 bread-starch exchange and 1 fat exchange
$\frac{1}{2}$ cup jello	1 bread-starch exchange
$\frac{1}{2}$ cup pudding	$\frac{1}{2}$ milk exchange and 1 bread-starch exchange
$\frac{1}{2}$ cup ice cream	1 bread-starch exchange and 2 fat exchanges
$\frac{1}{2}$ cup ice milk	1 bread-starch exchange and 1 fat exchange
$\frac{1}{4}$ cup sherbet	1 bread-starch exchange
3 ounces frozen yogurt	1 starch exchange, $\frac{1}{2}$ fruit exchange and 1 fat exchange

Evaluate Yourself 1

1. What is a free food?

2. Name five free foods.

3. What does dietetic mean?

4. What does the order of the list of ingredients tell you?

5. Here are two labels.
   a. Can you eat A and B?
   b. Do A and B contain sugar? What are they?
   c. If you can eat these foods, how much can you eat of them?

LABEL A	LABEL B
Serving size .... 2 sq.	Serving size .... 2 tsp.
Servings per cont. 5	Servings per container 30
Calories 81	Calories 14
Protein .... 2 gm.	Protein .... 0 gm.
Carbohydrate .... 7 gm.	Carbohydrate .... 3.5 gm.
Fat .... 5 gm.	Fat .... 0 gm.
Contains soybean oil, cocoa, sorbitol, milk solids, fructose, dextrins, preservatives	Contains corn syrup, sorbitol, water, preservatives

Answers to Evaluate Yourself 1

1. Free food is low in calories, protein, fat, and carbohydrate.

2. See the free food lists in this chapter.

3. Dietetic means one ingredient has been changed: calories, sugar, fat, salt, or cholesterol.

4. The ingredient in the largest amount on a product label is listed first.

5. a. A—no
      B—yes
   b. A—yes; fructose, dextrins, sorbitol
      B—yes; corn syrup, sorbitol
   c. A—none
      B—2 teaspoons

7
Putting It Together

MEASURE YOUR FOOD

The amount of food that you eat or drink tells you how much carbohydrate, protein, or fat you are eating. You must measure all your food until you can tell a serving by looking at it.

Here are some measurements that you will be using every day:

3 teaspoons equal **1 tablespoon**
16 tablespoons equal **1 cup**
48 teaspoons equal **1 cup**

8 ounces equal **1 cup**
4 ounces equal **½ cup**
16 ounces equal **1 pound**

2 cups equal **1 pint**
4 cups equal **1 quart**

You must keep these measurements in mind when you measure your food.

When you eat cooked foods, measure them after cooking. Keep in mind that meat, fish, and poultry shrink when they are cooked. These foods lose fat and water. For instance, when you cook four ounces of raw meat, you end up with three ounces of cooked meat. If you cook one pound of raw meat, you get twelve ounces of cooked meat.

Cut one pound of hamburger into quarters. Each quarter weighs 4 ounces. Freeze or package each quarter. When you cook one quarter, it will be 3 ounces of cooked meat.

Do not count the bone. You do not eat bone. Chicken and turkey are both 35 to 50 percent bone. If you buy a 3 pound chicken, count one-half of it as bone. One-quarter of a 2 to 3 pound chicken is about three ounces of cooked meat. The breast and wing have three ounces of meat. The thigh and leg have three ounces of meat.

Here are some ways to measure meat. You can use your hand to do this.

- Three ounces of cooked meat without bone is the size of a woman's hand (about 7 × 4 inches). And it is one-quarter inch thick, like this |__|

- Two ounces of cooked meat is the size of an average woman's palm. And it is one-quarter inch thick, like this |__|

- One ounce of cooked meat is the size of a woman's fingers. And it is one-quarter inch thick, like this

- You can use the cap of a 32 ounce jar of mayonnaise salad dressing to measure foods. This cap holds 3 ounces of cooked meat.

- You can use a scale. Keep in mind that:
   1 ounce equals 28 grams. (You can round this off to 30 grams.)
   2 ounces equals 56 grams. (You can round this off to 60 grams.)
   3 ounces equals 84 grams. (You can round this off to 90 grams)

- You can also use pictures. Compare Figure 7-2 to your serving of meat.

It is good to check the amount of food that you eat every once in awhile. Most of us will add a little bit extra here and there when we do not measure.

FOOD PREPARATION

We have talked about the amount of food that you can eat. Sometimes it is good to change the way that you cook a food to add flavor or variety, or to reduce calories. Here are some ideas you might want to try.

You can use foods that still have bulk in them, such as fiber, which make you feel more full. You can eat lettuce, carrot and celery sticks, fresh fruit, bran cereals, and other foods like these for bulk.

Use spices, herbs, fruit or vegetable juices, lemon juice, onion, vinegar, or wine to bring out the flavors in food. Use a spice chart to guide you. The alcohol in wine disappears in the cooking process and leaves a flavor. You will adjust to less rich food over a period of time.

You can use lean meats, fish, and cottage cheese. Trim the fat that you can see from the meat before you cook it. Rinse oil-packed fish, such as tuna, in water before you use it. Eat many kinds of breads to add variety to your meals.

You can eat many kinds of fruit. Eat fruit in place of dessert. Read the product label to make sure canned and frozen fruit does not have sugar added to it.

You may combine two vegetables for more variety. For instance, mix cauliflower with peas. Also, mix broccoli with mushrooms.

Read the label on skim milk. Make sure it contains vitamin A and vitamin D. You can use non-fat dry milk in cooking. This milk has fewer calories and fat than whole milk. This milk costs less too. Do *not* eat flavored yogurt as it contains added sugar. You can buy plain yogurt and add your own fruit.

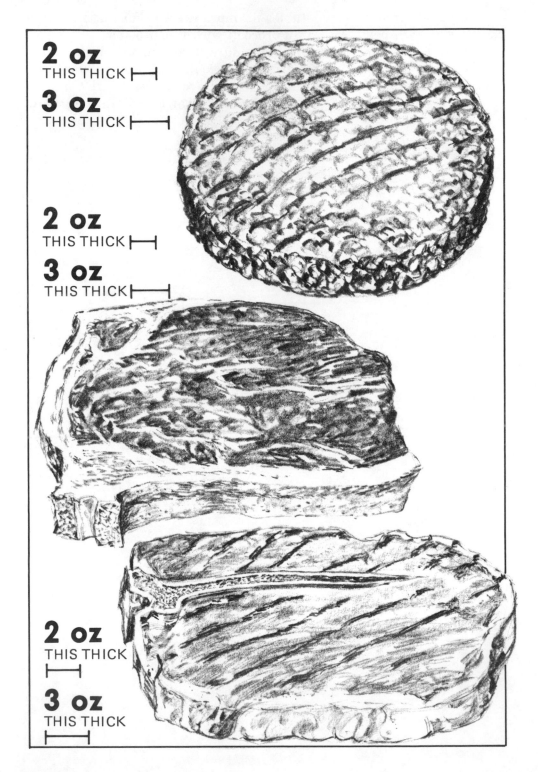

2 oz
THIS THICK |———|

3 oz
THIS THICK |————|

2 oz
THIS THICK |———|

3 oz
THIS THICK |————|

2 oz
THIS THICK
|———|

3 oz
THIS THICK
|————|

Figure 7-1.

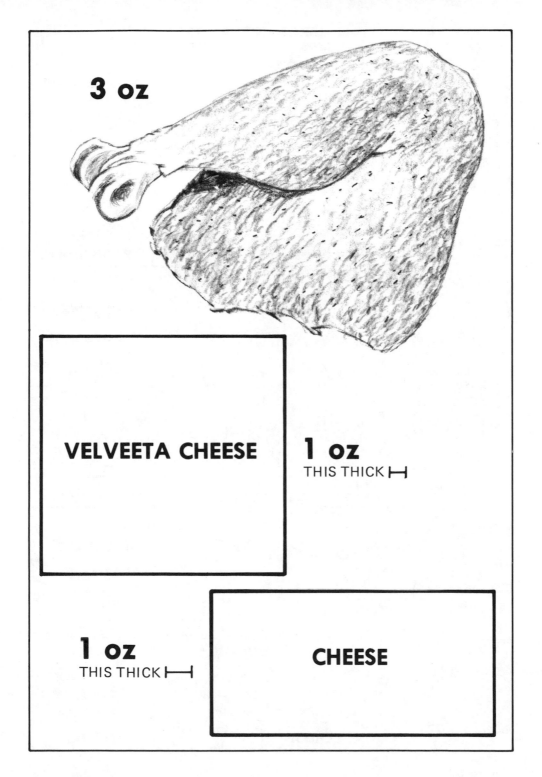

Figure 7-2.

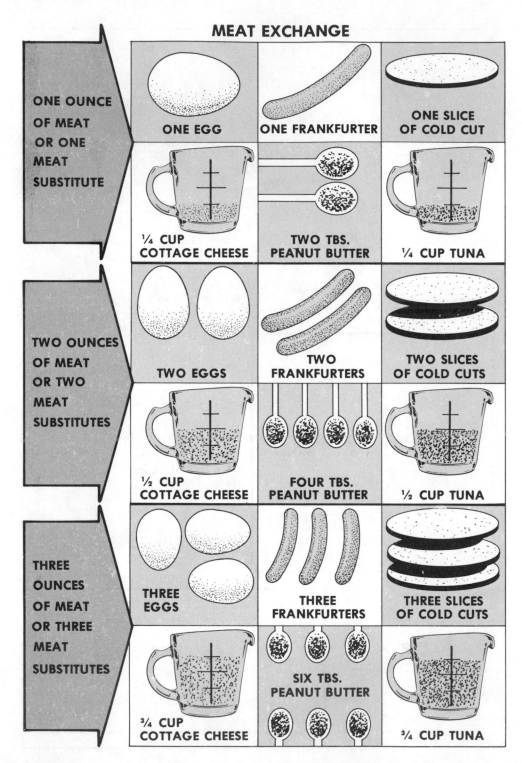

Figure 7-3.

8
Special Occasions

RESTAURANT CUISINE

There are times when you will eat in a restaurant. Or, you will have meals that have been prepared by someone else. You can enjoy eating out. Below are some hints that are good to keep in mind.

Know your meal plan, and your food exchanges from each food group. You may want to carry a copy of your plan in your purse or wallet. Eat a snack if you are going to eat later than normal. You can eat your fruit or milk choice for a snack instead of having this at dinner. Or, you can eat your evening snack at your dinner hour. Then eat your dinner at your snack time.

Many restaurants do not serve cooked vegetables. You can eat an extra ½ bread-starch exchange in place of one vegetable serving. You can save up all of your fat exchanges from the whole day. You can eat all of them at one meal.

You can save one or two meat exchanges from your other meals. Then add these meat exchanges to your evening meal.

Ask your waitress or chef about the portion size, how the food is cooked and what food items have been added to a dish. Restaurants do not list all available items on the menu. You can ask for skim milk, margarine, and main entrees without gravy or sauces. Ask your waitress to serve salad dressings, gravy, margarine, and sour cream on the side. You can then add the amount that you want to.

You can eat most foods that are served in a restaurant. There are foods that are better food choices than others. Some of these foods are listed below.

Appetizers: Use "free" vegetables, clear broths, consomme, or dill pickles.

Meat, fish, chicken: Eat broiled, baked, roasted, or boiled meat, poultry, and fish. Trim off all visible fat. BEWARE: Some restaurants will add fat to meat or fish before broiling.

Eggs: Order soft or hard boiled, poached or baked.

Potatoes: Order baked, boiled, or mashed.

Vegetables: Order steamed, baked, boiled, or stewed vegetables.

Salads: Use lemon juice, vinegar, or low calorie salad dressing for your vegetable salad.

Fruit: Eat fresh fruit, fresh fruit salad, or unsweetened fruit juice.

Breads: Order breads that are not frosted or glazed. For variety, you can order hard or soft dinner rolls, plain muffins, biscuits, crackers, or popovers.

Fats: Use butter, margarine, salad dressing, gravy, bacon, cream, oil, olives, or nuts.

Desserts: Ask for fresh fruits or unsweetened canned fruits. Some restaurants do have these items.

Beverages: Drink coffee, decaffeinated coffee, tea, sugar-free soft drink, or milk.

When you choose other foods, you will be eating hidden fat, sugar, and calories. You then have to give up some extra food exchanges.

Here are some foods you can eat and the exchanges you will have to give up to eat them.

- Buttered vegetables: omit one fat exchange for each ½ cup serving of vegetable.
- Fried foods: omit two fat exchanges for each exchange of meat, fish, or chicken.
- Cream sauces: do not eat all of the sauce. Omit one or two fat exchanges.
- Foods that already have a dressing mixed in them: Omit one fat exchange for each ½ cup exchange.
- Meat or fish appetizers and cottage cheese: You cannot eat as much meat with your entree if you eat these.
- Desserts: See your dessert list.
- Do not drink chocolate milk or cocoa.

Fast Foods

You may also choose to eat at a fast food restaurant. Ask your dietitian for an exchange list.

ALCOHOLIC BEVERAGES

There may be times when you want to drink alcohol. You can drink alcohol safely. First, talk this over with your doctor. Your doctor will tell you how much you may drink, and how often it may be okay to drink alcohol. Keep these facts in mind, if your doctor permits the use of alcohol.

- *Alcohol lowers your blood sugar.* You can have an insulin reaction if you drink too much alcohol, or if you have not eaten for a while. Your insulin reaction could come at any time. You could be driving a car, sleeping, or at a party.

- *The right time for you to drink alcohol is right before or after eating.* Eating will raise your blood sugar. Eat food right after you have a drink. Or, you can have an after-dinner drink.

- *Alcohol is high in calories.* One gram of alcohol has 7 calories. One ounce of liquor has about 90 calories.

The chart below shows you how to substitute alcohol for other foods in your meal plan.

Alcoholic beverages	Food group
• 12 ounces of beer	1 bread-starch exchange and 2 fat exchanges
• 12 ounces of light beer	2 fat exchanges
• 3½ ounces dry wine	½ bread-starch exchange and ½ fat exchange
• 2 ounces dry sherry	½ bread-starch exchange and 2 fat exchanges
• 1 ounce gin, rum, vodka, whiskey	2 fat exchanges

Here are some points to keep in mind when you drink alcohol. Do not drink more than:

2 exchanges of gin, rum, vodka or whiskey; or
1 exchange of beer; or
1 exchange of dry wine; or
1 exchange of dry sherry.

Do not drink this amount more than three or four times a week. If you use a mix, use:

sugar-free soft drink, pop, or soda

tomato juice
club soda
water
orange juice

Keep in mind that orange juice is a fruit exchange. You can drink beer or wine instead of bread-starch and fat exchanges. The reason for this is that beer and wine contain carbohydrate. The calories from the pure alcohol are substituted for fat. Do not give up other foods to drink alcohol.

MENU PLANNING

Plan a meal that you would order in a restaurant. Also, plan your other meals and snacks for the day.

BREAKFAST

_____ fruit exchange
_____ meat exchange
_____ bread–starch exchange

_____ fat exchange
_____ cup(s) of milk

LUNCH

_____ meat exchange
_____ bread–starch exchange

_____ vegetable exchange
_____ vegetable exchange
_____ fruit exchange
_____ fat exchange
_____ cup(s) of milk

DINNER

_____ meat exchange
_____ bread–starch exchange

_____ vegetable exchange
_____ vegetable exchange

———— fruit exchange
———— fat exchange
———— cup(s) of milk

SNACKS

Morning   Afternoon   Evening

Evaluate Yourself 1

1. When is the best time to drink alcohol?

2. Why is it important not to drink alcohol on an empty stomach?

3. What kind of food will raise your blood sugar the most when you drink alcohol?

4. Name some foods that are good to eat or drink before you drink alcohol.

5. Will peanuts make your blood sugar rise?

6. How many servings of alcohol can you drink at one time?

7. Name the beverages that you can mix with alcohol.

8. What can you do if you are going to eat later than usual?

9. What are two foods that have the least effect on your blood sugar right away?

Answers to Evaluate Yourself 1

1. Drink alcohol right before or right after a meal.
2. Alcohol makes your blood sugar fall. When you have not eaten for 2 to 4 hours, your blood sugar is also falling.
3. Carbohydrate raises your blood sugar the most when drinking alcohol.
4. Milk, fruit, and bread-starch foods, such as crackers, bread, popcorn, and potato chips are good to eat before drinking alcohol.
5. No, peanuts are a fat food. Fat does not raise your blood sugar very much.
6. Drink moderate amounts. Each person can tolerate a different amount. It is a good idea to limit your intake to about 2 servings of gin, rum, vodka, or one serving of either beer or wine. Keep in mind the high caloric content of alcohol.
7. Mix tomato juice, club soda, water, or orange juice with alcohol.
8. Eat your snack at meal time and your meal at snack time. Eat a small serving of food that has carbohydrate in it. Eat your fruit or milk serving from your meal.
9. Meat and fat. Meat contains protein and does not affect your blood sugar as much as carbohydrate. Fat contains only fat and hardly affects your blood sugar. But keep in mind, both protein and fat still add calories.

9
Illness

MENU PLANNING FOR ILLNESS

There may be days when you are not able to eat as you usually do. You may have the flu with nausea and vomiting. You may have a sore mouth from dental work. Or, you may have a bad cold with a fever. If your illness is short term, you may have to change your meal plan. Eat those foods that best agree with you. If your illness lasts *longer* than one day, call your doctor.

When you are ill, you must:

- Take your insulin or oral hypoglycemic pills.
- Check your urine or blood sugar at least four times for sugar.
- Check your urine for ketones.
- Eat some form of food that contains carbohydrates.
- Eat small meals many times a day. Eat at least six times a day or every one to two hours.

During illness, it is *best* to eat carbohydrate foods. Remember, carbohydrate foods have the most effect on your blood sugar. When you are ill you also need extra calories and other nutrients.

What can you eat or drink when you are sick? Here is a list of foods you can eat instead of milk, fruit, vegetables, and bread-starches. Some of the foods on the list are eaten *only* when you are ill. These foods are high in sugar and low in all other nutrients. Eat or drink about 4 ounces (½ cup) of these high sugar foods at a time. Do *not* drink a 12 ounce can of soft drink in one hour. Drink 4 ounces of the soft drink an hour. You do *not* have to replace foods from the meat and fat groups.

Food Exchanges

Milk list: You can eat these foods instead of one cup of milk.

eggnog	1 cup
cream soup	1 cup
chocolate milk	1 cup (omit 1 bread-starch exchange)
custard	½ cup (omit 1 fruit exchange)
plain yogurt	½ cup

Starch list: You can eat these foods instead of one bread-starch exchange.

bread or toast	1 slice
ice cream	½ cup
sherbet	¼ cup
cooked cereal	½ cup
saltines	6
soup—noodle or starchy	1 cup
regular jello	½ cup
instant breakfast	½ cup
carbonated beverage, regular	1 cup

Fruit list: You can eat these foods instead of one fruit exchange.

apple, apricot or pineapple juice, pear or peach nectar	⅓ cup
prune or grape juice	¼ cup
orange or grapefruit juice	½ cup
twin popsicle	½
carbonated beverage, regular	½ cup
honey	2 teaspoons
sugar	2½ teaspoons
regular jello	¼ cup

You can eat ½ serving of bread-starch exchange instead of ½ cup of vegetable.

Add Up Your Carbohydrate

Know how many exchanges of milk, vegetable, fruit, and bread-starch are in each meal and snack of your meal plan. You can write them here.

Breakfast

Snack

Lunch

Snack

Dinner

Snack

MENU PLANNING

Plan one day's food intake for when you are sick.
Meal one at_____(time)

Meal two at_____(time)

Meal three at_____(time)

Meal four at_____(time)

Meal five at_____(time)

Meal six at_____(time)

Evaluate Yourself 1

1. Should you take your insulin or pills when you are sick?

2. Should you test your urine more often when you are sick?
   _____ How often?

3. When should you call your doctor?

4. Why is it important to eat when you are sick?

5. What kinds of food should you eat?

6. How often should you eat or drink?

Answers to Evaluate Yourself 1

1. Yes, you must take your insulin or pills when you are sick.
2. Yes; you must test your urine or blood sugar at least four times a day.
3. If your urine is ½%, 1%, or 2% for two days, or your urine is ½%, 1%, or 2% with ketones, you must call your doctor.
4. Your body needs sugar all day long even when you are sick. When you are ill you also need extra calories and other nutrients.
5. You must eat carbohydrate foods like milk, fruit, vegetables, and bread-starch exchanges or sugar foods when you are sick.
6. When you are sick, you must eat 6–8 times a day, or every 1–2 hours.

10
Potpourri

THIS 'N THAT MEALS

A lot of the foods that you eat are a mixture of foods. When you eat a casserole or other type of hot dish, you are eating two, three, or even four kinds of food. If you eat a lot of these meals, here is how you can save some time.

You do not have to figure out some recipes each time that you make them. You can use a general recipe that will be close enough.

You can make a hot dish, a casserole, stew, chili, or macaroni and cheese. In making one of these dishes, you are eating:

- STARCH: The starch exchanges are in the noodles, vegetables, potato, rice, or chili beans.
- MEAT: The meat exchanges are hamburger, tuna, chicken, beef, or cheese.
- FAT: The fat exchanges are cream soups, gravy, or a cream sauce.

One cup of any of these dishes is like eating:
  2 meat exchanges
  1 bread-starch exchange
  and 1 fat exchange.
This 'n that meals include the Chinese, Mexican, and Italian meals shown below.

Chinese

One cup of chow mein or chop suey is like eating 1 vegetable exchange and 1–2 meat exchanges. One-half cup of Chinese noodles is equal to 1 bread-starch exchange and 1 fat exchange. One-half cup of rice is equal to 1 bread-starch exchange.

Italian

Pizza is a food that can be eaten at any mealtime. The crust of a pizza is a *starch* exchange. The tomato sauce is a *fat* exchange. Mushrooms, green pepper, tomato, and onion are *vegetable* exchanges. The hamburger, pepperoni, sausage, cheese, and shrimp garnishes are *meat* exchanges.

The amount of each food group on the pizza depends on the kind of pizza. Was the pizza frozen? Did you buy the pizza at a restaurant? Did you make the pizza? Is it a deep dish pizza? The amount of meat exchanges depends on the amount of meat and cheese that is on the pizza. Ask your dietitian for an exchange list that gives you the exchanges for pizza houses in your area and commercial pizzas.

Here are some guidelines for eating pizza and what each exchange contains.

One-twelfth of a 10-inch frozen meat pizza is like eating:
1 bread-starch exchange
1–2 meat exchanges
0–1 fat exchange.

One-sixth of an 8 × 9 inch frozen deep dish pizza is like eating:

2 bread-starch exchanges
1–2 meat exchanges
0–1 fat exchange.

You can eat an Italian spaghetti dinner too. One-half cup spaghetti noodles is 1 bread-starch exchange. One cup of tomato sauce is like eating 1 bread-starch exchange and 1 fat exchange. One cup of tomato sauce with meat added is like eating:

1 bread-starch exchange
1–2 meat exchanges
2 fat exchanges.

One cooked meatball one inch round equals one meat exchange (1 oz).

Mexican

Mexican foods can add spice to your life. The spices used are thought of as free foods.

This is how you plan to include some Mexican foods into your meal plan.

One taco is like eating 2 meat exchanges and 1 bread-starch exchange. A beef enchilada with cheese sauce is like eating 1 bread-starch exchange and 2 meat exchanges. A bean enchilada is like eating 2 bread-starch exchanges and 1 meat exchange.

Soup

Soups are mixtures of milk, vegetables, bread-starch, meats, and fats. Most soups contain a small amount of milk, meat, and fat that we will not count. In order to make it easier for you, you can eat soup instead of either vegetable or bread-starch foods.

One cup of vegetable soup is like eating 1 *vegetable* exchange. One cup of any other soup is like eating 1 *bread-starch* exchange. If you want a soup exchange list, ask your dietitian for one.

Ask your dietitian to help you with any special recipes. She or he can give you extra lists for many foods. You can also use diabetic cookbooks. A list of cookbooks is shown below.

FOOD-FOR-THOUGHT

Cookbooks for Diabetic Diets

The Calculating Cook (200 recipes)
Written by Jeanne Jones
Price: $5.00   1972

Recipes from sauces to desserts. A lot of the recipes use gourmet cookery and can add spice to your eating.

Diet for a Happy Heart (170 recipes)
Written by Jeanne Jones
Price: $5.00 1975

A cookbook that combines the diabetic diet and a low cholesterol diet. Again, Jeanne Jones uses the art of gourmet cookery.

Diabetes Control Cookery (155 recipes)
Written by Dorothy Revell
1621 S. University Drive
Fargo, ND 58103
Price: $2.25 (5 cents state tax added) (postage 25 cents) 1975

A cookbook for the experienced cook that includes food charts, food during illness, exchange values of commonly used ingredients, and a guide for calculating your recipes into exchanges.

Diet Delight Cookbook for Diabetic Children
Written by Jeanne Jones
California Canners and Growers
Cookbook Department
3100 Ferry Building
San Francisco, CA 94106

Exchange Lists for Meal Planning
Written by American Diabetes Association
2 Park Avenue
New York, New York 10016
Price: 75 cents
How to use exchanges to vary the diet.

The American Diabetes Association/American Dietetic Association Family Cookbook (250 recipes)
Price: $12.95 plus $2.50 for postage and handling
Available from The American Diabetes Association
2 Park Avenue
New York, New York 10016
Also available from your local American Diabetes Association chapter.

This book features more than 250 delicious, economical, kitchen-tested recipes the whole family will savor; an exchange equivalents and nutrients per serving guide for each recipe; important tips on eating out and brown-bagging it, weight control, exercise, and much more. For diabetics, it is an encyclopedia of nutrition how-to's ranging from the use of these recipes in daily meal plans to balancing food and medication during sick days.

RECIPE EXCHANGE

You can adapt your own favorite recipe by the method shown here.

1. List all the ingredients in the recipe you are using. List the amount of each ingredient used in the recipe.
2. Identify the exchange group that each ingredient is found in. Record the total number of exchanges in each ingredient. Keep in mind that cooked and uncooked amounts are a different number of food exchanges.

The exchange for a cooked food may not be the same as the exchange for a raw food. The exchange changes because the food can increase or decrease in size. For instance, rice doubles in size when you cook it. It becomes moist and expands.

3. Add up the total number of exchanges from each food group.
4. Divide the total number of exchanges for each food group by the total number of servings. Round off to the nearest one-half exchange. Do not count anything less than one-half exchange.

Here is one example of a recipe exchange for peanut butter cookies. The recipe makes four dozen (48) cookies. Each of the steps in the list above is numbered in the example below.

PEANUT BUTTER COOKIES

1. Cream and blend ½ cup butter, ½ cup peanut butter, ⅓ cup sugar, ⅓ cup brown sugar, 1 egg, and 1 tsp vanilla in a mixing bowl.
2. Sift together the dry ingredients: 1¼ cup sifted flour, ¾ tsp baking soda, and ¼ tsp salt.
3. Blend the dry ingredients into the creamed mixture.
4. Shape the mixture into one-inch balls.
5. Roll the balls in granulated sugar.
6. Place two inches apart on an ungreased cookie sheet.
7. Bake at 375° Fahrenheit for 10–12 minutes. Makes four dozen cookies.

- One peanut butter cookie is like eating:
  ½ fruit exchange
  ¼ bread-starch exchange
  ½ fat exchange
- Two cookies are like eating:
  1 fruit exchange
  ½ bread-starch exchange
  1 fat exchange

Table 10–1. Ingredients and Exchange Groups in Peanut Butter Cookies.

1. INGREDIENTS	2. EXCHANGE GROUPS						
	Milk	Fruit	Vegetable	Bread-starch	Meat	Fat	Free
½ cup butter						18	
½ cup peanut butter				1½	4	18	
1¼ cup flour				8½			
⅓ cup brown sugar		4½					
⅓ cup sugar		7					
¾ tsp soda							X
¼ tsp salt							X
½ tsp vanilla							X
3. TOTAL EXCHANGES	0	11½	0	10	4	36	0
4. TOTAL EXCHANGES / TOTAL SERVINGS = EXCHANGE PER SERVING	0	$\frac{11½}{48}$	0	$\frac{10}{48}$	$\frac{4}{48}$	$\frac{36}{48}$	0
4. ROUND OFF		¼		¼	⅑	¾	0

Here is a blank form for you to use to adapt your own recipes.

Table 10–2. Sample Form to List Your Favorite Recipe Ingredients and Exchange Groups.

1. INGREDIENTS	2. EXCHANGE GROUPS						
	Milk	Fruit	Vegetable	Bread-starch	Meat	Fat	Free
3. TOTAL EXCHANGES							
4. TOTAL EXCHANGES TOTAL SERVINGS = EXCHANGE PER SERVING							
4. ROUND OFF							

MASS MEASUREMENTS FOR RECIPES AND THEIR EXCHANGE VALUES

The figures that were used to translate the nutrient content of a certain food into exchanges were obtained from Agricultural Handbook No. 456 from the USDA.

Foods high in sugar are translated into fruit exchanges. The only food exchange group that contains carbohydrate is the fruit group. Sugar is 100 percent carbohydrate. Keep in mind that the high sugar foods lack vitamins and minerals.

When a large amount of a food is translated into an exchange, you may notice that the exchanges used do not seem to match the kind of food. This is due to the fact that a large number of foods contain small amounts of a nutrient—carbohydrate, protein, or fat. These small amounts are taken into account when the translation is made.

Fruit

Apricots, dried halves, one pound: 13½ fruit
Figs, one 2½ inch: 1 fruit
Prunes, 1 cup without pits: 12 fruit
Cranberries, 1 cup, raw: 1 fruit
Raisins, 1 cup: 11 fruit
Pumpkin, 1 cup: 2 bread-starch
Lemon juice, 1 cup: 2 fruit
Dates, 1 cup, chopped: 13 fruit

Sugar

1 cup brown, packed: 21 fruit
1 cup brown: 14 fruit
1 cup granulated: 20 fruit
1 cup powdered: 10 fruit
Marshmallow
2 large: 1 fruit
1 cup miniature: 4 fruit
Candied cherries
4 oz (¾ cup): 10 fruit
10: 3 fruit
Honey, 1 cup: 28 fruit
Molasses, 1 cup: 21 fruit
Cocoa, plain, 1 cup: 4 fruit, 2 meat, 1 fat
1 tbsp: ⅓ fruit
Chocolate syrup, 1 cup: 19 fruit, 1 meat
Maple syrup, 1 cup: 20½ fruit
1 tbsp: 1 fruit
Corn syrup, 1 cup: 24½ fruit
1 tbsp: 1½ fruit

Starch

Rice, 1 cup dry: 11 bread-starch
Macaroni, one pound dry: 23 bread-starch
Egg noodles, one pound dry: 2 bread-starch, 2 meat, 2 fat
Cornstarch, 1 cup dry: 11 fruit
1 tbsp: ¾ fruit
Tapioca, 1 cup dry: 13 fruit
Barley, 1 cup dry: 10 bread-starch
Flour, 1 cup, unsifted: 7 bread-starch
1 cup sifted: 6 bread-starch
1 tbsp: ½ bread-starch
Cake flour, 1 cup unsifted: 5 bread-starch
1 cup sifted: 5 bread-starch

Soup

Cream of chicken soup, 1 can: ½ fruit, 2 meat, medium-fat, 2 fat
Cream of mushroom soup, 1 can: ½ fruit, 3 meat, medium-fat, 2 fat

Vegetable

Whole canned tomatoes, 16 oz: 4 vegetable
Tomato paste, 6 oz: 2 bread-starch
Tomato puree, 29 oz: 5 bread-starch

Milk

Milk, 1 cup evaporated: 2 cups regular milk, or
                         2 cups skim milk, 4 fat
      1 cup condensed: 3 cups skim milk: 13 fruit,
                   5½ fat or 3 cups 2% milk, 13 fruit, 2 fat

Meat Substitutes

Egg, one white: ½ meat, medium-fat, subtract 1 fat
  one yolk: ½ meat, medium-fat, 1 fat
Peanut butter, 1 cup: 3 bread-starch, 8 meat, medium-fat, 18 fat

Fat

Butter, ½ cup (4 oz): 18 fat
Margarine, 1 cup: 2 bread-starch, 37 fat
Mayonnaise, 1 cup: 35 fat
Mayonnaise Salad Dressing, 1 cup: 3½ fruit, 20 fat
Cream cheese, 8 oz: ½ fruit, 2½ meat, medium-fat, 15 fat
Cream, half and half, 1 cup: 1 fruit, 1 meat, medium-fat, 4½ fat
  light, 1 cup: 1 fruit, 1 meat, medium-fat, 9 fat
  whipping, 1 cup (2 cups whipped): 1 fruit, 1 meat, medium-fat, 14 fat
  heavy, 1 cup: ¾ fruit, ½ meat, medium-fat, 17 fat
Coconut, 1 cup packed: 1 fruit, ½ meat, medium-fat, 8 fat
  1 cup: ½ bread-starch, 6 fat
Vegetable oil, 1 cup: 40 fat
Lard, 1 cup: 41 fat
  1 tbsp: 2½ fat

Nuts

Walnuts, 1 cup: 1 bread-starch, 3 meat, medium-fat, 12 fat
  1 cup ground: 1 fruit, 2 meat, medium-fat, 7 fat
Slivered almonds, 1 cup: 2 fruit, 3 meat, medium-fat, 10 fat
Almonds, one pound: 1 fruit, 5 bread-starch, 11 meat, medium-fat, 38 fat
Cashews, 1 cup: 4 fruit, 3½ meat, medium-fat, 9 fat

Spanish peanuts, one pound: 5½ bread-starch, 16 meat, medium-fat, 27
   fat
   1 cup: 2 bread-starch, 4½ meat, medium-fat, 10 fat
Pecans, 1 cup: 1 bread-starch, 1 meat, medium-fat, 14 fat

Miscellaneous

Yeast: free food exchange
Baking powder: free food exchange
Cream of tartar: free food exchange

LABELS DO TELL

When you buy a box of macaroni and cheese, do you know how much
cheese you will be eating? How do you plan one serving of this into your
meal plan? If you read the label, you can find out.

All labels must tell you the

- brand name,
- product name,
- manufacturer's address,
- amount of food in the package or the net weight.

Many products will give you nutritional information. Products that
make a nutritional claim must give you this information. Other products
will give you this information even though they do not make a nutritional
claim.
   When manufacturers make a nutritional claim, they are saying that
their product is different from the normal food product. The product
could be low in calories, low in sugar, or low in salt. It could also be low in
fat or other ingredients.
   The label on a product must tell you the

- total number of servings
- size of the serving
- number of calories per serving
- amount of carbohydrate in grams
- amount of protein in grams
- amount of fat in grams

The amount of carbohydrate, protein, and fat in the product is written in
grams. If the product claims that it is low in salt or any other nutrient,
the amount per serving must also be listed.
   You will see some other nutrients listed on a product. These are
protein, vitamin A, vitamin C, thiamin, riboflavin, niacin, calcium, and

iron. The label does not tell you the amount of a nutrient that is in the product but does tell you the percentage of the nutrient that you are getting in one serving. The label does not tell you what the needs are for a child, a pregnant woman, or a sick person.

The daily nutrient needs of healthy people in the United States are called the Recommended Daily Dietary Allowances. You will see these allowances written like this on food labels—U.S. RDA.

For instance, a label can say, "Iron . . . 10". This means that you are eating 10 percent of the iron that you need for one day. Keep in mind that you are eating 10 percent of your iron needs in *one serving*.

How can you use food labels to plan a food product into your meal plan? First, you have to know the nutrients that are in each food group. Each food group has a certain number of grams of carbohydrate, protein, and fat in *one exchange*. These groups and their composition are listed below.

Table 10-3. Nutrient Content of Exchanges.

	Carbohydrate grams	Protein grams	Fat grams
1 cup skim milk	12	8	0
1 cup 2% milk	12	8	5
1 cup regular milk	12	8	10
1 vegetable exchange	5	2	0
1 fruit exchange	10	0	0
1 bread-starch exchange	15	2	0
1 meat exchange, low fat	0	7	3
1 meat exchange, medium fat	0	7	5
1 meat exchange, high fat	0	7	7
1 fat exchange	0	0	5

Ask yourself: Is the product you are going to eat a bread-starch food, a fruit, a vegetable, or a meat food? Look at the first two or three ingredients. Use the list of ingredients to help you choose a food group. For instance, if milk is listed first, choose a milk exchange.

Here are some things to keep in mind as you add up the food exchanges in your product.

- Your total for each of the three nutrients must be within *3 grams* of what is printed on the label. It can be 1–3 grams more, or it can be 1–3 grams less. Most of the time, your total nutrient content will not be the same as what is listed on the label. But you will be close.
- Try not to use a half-exchange from a food group.
- Begin with the food groups that contain carbohydrate. These food groups are the milk, fruit, vegetable, and bread-starch groups. Figure the food group with protein in it next, then the meat group. Plan the fat group last.
- You can round off a fraction to the next whole number.

Let's use the label on a box of macaroni and cheese. The exchange size is ¾ cup cooked. The total number of grams in *one exchange* is:

30 grams of carbohydrate,
 8 grams of protein,
13 grams of fat.

These numbers are our goal.

The food ingredients are listed in this order: macaroni, cheese, and then milk. Macaroni is the first ingredient and is in the bread-starch group. So, you will choose exchanges from the bread-starch group first. Let's begin.

	(CHO) Carbohydrate grams	Protein grams	Fat grams
1. Your goal is:	30	8	13
2. Look at your nutrient chart.			
3. One bread-starch exchange contains 15 grams of CHO and 2 grams of protein. *Two bread-starch* exchanges contain 30 grams of CHO, and 4 grams of protein.	30	4	0
4. You have this amount left over.	0	4	13

	(CHO) Carbohydrate	Protein	Fat
5. The food group that contains protein and fat is the meat group.			
One exchange of meat contains 7 grams of protein and 5 grams of fat.			
One-half exchange of medium fat meat contains 3.5 grams of protein and 2.5 grams of fat.			
Round off to 4 grams of	0	4	13
protein and 3 grams of fat.	0	4	3
6. Subtract from your subtotal.			
7. You have this amount left over.	0	0	10
8. The only food group with fat in it is the fat group.	0	0	10
One fat exchange contains 5 grams of fat.			
Two fat exchanges contain 10 grams of fat.	0	0	10
9. Subtract from your subtotal.			
You do not have any nutrients left over.	0	0	0
Let's review.			
One exchange contains	30	8	13
We have planned 2 bread-starch exchanges			
½ meat exchange, medium fat 2 fat exchanges			
This is a total of	30	8	13
The difference is	0	0	0

Let's do another product: a vegetable soup. The exchange size is 10 ounces. The total number of grams in *one exchange* is

22 grams of carbohydrate (CHO),
3 grams of protein,
4 grams of fat.

These numbers are our goal.

The food ingredients of the soup are listed in this order: water, carrots, potato, celery, zucchini, tomato, corn, lima beans, green beans, peas, potato starch, vegetable oil, cabbage, sugar, vegetable protein, and sweet red peppers. Vegetables are the main ingredients, so you will use vegetable exchanges first.

	(CHO) Carbohydrate	Protein	Fat
1. Our goal is:	22	3	4
2. Look at your nutrient chart.			
3. 1 vegetable exchange contains 5 grams CHO, 2 grams protein. 2 vegetable exchanges contain 10 grams CHO, 4 grams protein. 3 vegetable exchanges contain 15 grams CHO, 6 grams protein. You have planned too much extra protein. So, you will choose *2 vegetable exchanges.*	10	4	0
4. Subtract from your goal. You have planned for 1 gram of protein too much, but it is not more than 3 grams.	12	1 too much	4
5. You have 12 grams of CHO left. The only food group that contains CHO is the fruit group. *One fruit exchange* contains 10 grams CHO.	10	0	0
6. Subtract from subtotal.	2	1 too much	4

	(CHO) Carbohydrate	Protein	Fat

7. You have not planned for 2 grams CHO. It is less than 3 grams.

8. The only food group with fat in it is fat.

   1 fat exchange contains 5 grams fat.

	0	0	5

9. Subtract from your total. You have planned one extra gram of fat, which is too much, but it is less than 3 grams.

		1 too much	

   You do not count the 2 grams of carbohydrate, 1 gram protein and 1 gram fat.

Let's review

One Exchange contains

	22	3	4

We have planned
   2 vegetable exchanges
   1 fruit exchange
   1 fat exchange

This is a total of:

	20	4	5

The difference is:

	2	1	1

It is less than 3 grams
for each nutrient.

The calories on *the soup label* are:
   22 grams CHO × 4 calories/gram   =   88 calories
   3 grams protein × 4 calories/gram   =   12 calories
   4 grams fat × 9 calories/gram   =   36 calories

   The total is: 136 calories

The calories on *your plan* are:
   20 grams CHO × 4 calories/gram   =   80 calories
   4 grams protein × 4 calories/gram   =   16 calories
   5 grams fat × 9 calories/gram   =   45 calories

   The total is: 141 calories

There is a difference of only 5 calories.

Here is another way we could plan the soup.

	(CHO) Carbohydrate	Protein	Fat
1. Your goal is:	22	3	2
2. Your product contains potato. Potato is in the bread-starch group. One bread-starch exchange contains 15 grams CHO, 2 grams protein.	15	2	0
3. Subtract from your goal.			
4. You have this amount left over.	7	1	4
5. The food group that contains about 7 grams CHO and 1 gram protein is the vegetable group.	7	1	4
One vegetable exchange contains 5 grams CHO, 2 grams protein.	5	2	0
6. Subtract from your subtotal.	2	1 too much	4
7. You have planned one gram of protein too much. We have 2 grams CHO left over. They are less than 3 grams each.			
8. The only food group with fat in it is fat.			
One fat exchange contains 5 grams fat.	0	0	5
9. Subtract from your subtotal. You have planned 1 gram of fat too much. But it is less than 3 grams.		1 too much	

Let's review.

One exchange contains:	22	3	4

You have planned
  1 bread-starch exchange
  1 vegetable exchange
  1 fat exchange

	(CHO) Carbohydrate	Protein	Fat
This is a total of:	20	4	5
The difference is:	2	1	1

The difference is less than 3 grams
for each nutrient.

The calories on *the label* are:

22 grams CHO × 4 calories/gram	=	88 calories
3 grams protein × 4 calories/gram	=	12 calories
4 grams fat × 9 calories/gram	=	36 calories
The total is:		136 calories

The calories on *your plan* are:

20 grams CHO × 4 calories/gram	=	80 calories
4 grams protein × 4 calories/gram	=	16 calories
5 grams fat × 9 calories/gram	=	45 calories
The total is:		141 calories

There is a difference of only 5 calories.

PLAN YOUR LABEL

You can use this form to adapt the exchanges in one serving of a purchased food.

	(CHO) Carbohydrate	Protein	Fat
1. The total grams on the label			
2. CHO foods—read the list of ingredients.			
3. Protein foods			
4. Fat foods			

11
From Head To Toe

DIABETES COMPLICATIONS

Diabetes is a lifelong partner. In order for you to enjoy good health you must control your diabetes.

Diabetes is not a simple disease—it can affect your body in many ways. These effects are called the complications of diabetes. One of the reasons you control diabetes is to avoid or delay these complications. Recent research seems to indicate near normal blood sugar control (70–140 mgm %) can prevent or minimize complications. The complications include:

1. *Changes in the blood vessels.* A diabetic's blood vessels seem to age faster than those of a nondiabetic. When blood vessels age:
   A. The walls of the vessels become less elastic. They are not able to pump blood with such great force. The result is: The rate and amount of blood flow (circulation) is decreased.
   B. The inside walls of the vessels begin to pick up fatty deposits or fatty debris. This can decrease the space for blood to flow through. The result is: A smaller amount of blood is carried throughout the body.

2. *Changes in the Nerves.* This change in the nerves is called diabetic neuropathy. Symptoms of nerve damage are tingling, numbness in your feet or hands, and pain. Also, you may not be able to feel heat or cold on your legs, toes, or fingers. Nerve damage can also cause sexual problems. Scientists are not certain what causes nerve damage in diabetes. They think it is related to high blood sugar harming the nerve cells.

3. *Infections.* Diabetics tend to be more prone to some infections. Their bodies may not be able to fight infection as well or as quickly as that of a nondiabetic.

What can you do to stay healthy? First, *control your blood sugar.* Second, *be alert to the parts of your body that the complications affect.* The small blood vessels carry blood to your kidneys, eyes, and mouth.

The Kidneys

1. Protect your kidneys by drinking plenty of fluids daily. (Eight cups of fluid are recommended.)
2. Infections can move from the bladder to the kidneys. Promptly report any of the following signs of a bladder infection to your doctor:
   - painful or burning urination
   - it is hard to empty your bladder
   - blood in the urine
   - pus in the urine
   - need to urinate more often.

The Eyes

1. Visit an opthalmologist at least once a year. Tell him or her that you have diabetes. An opthalmologist is a doctor who is an expert on the eyes. Optometrists or opticians are experts in fitting glasses or grinding lenses.
2. If your vision becomes blurry, check your urine or blood tests. One cause of blurred vision is high blood sugar. Report blurred vision to your doctor if it persists.

The Mouth

1. Visit a dentist twice a year. Remind him or her that you have diabetes. A dentist will pay special attention to the gum tissue. Gum tissue supports the teeth. This tissue can be harmed by poor circulation and uncontrolled diabetes.
2. Your dentist will teach you proper flossing and brushing of your teeth. This will help prevent gum infection and dental decay. Your diet will help also!
3. If you wear dentures, check your mouth daily with a mirror. Look for red spots, sores, or cuts. Promptly report these to your dentist. They can become infected.

The large blood vessels carry blood to your heart, legs, and feet.

The Heart

1. Follow your diabetic diet. The meal plan is designed to reduce the amount of those foods that may be related to heart disease. The diet

is also designed to help you achieve ideal body weight. Being over-weight increases the work your heart must do.

2. Avoid smoking. Smoking constricts (narrows) blood vessels and thereby reduces blood flow. Smokers have a higher incidence of heart disease than nonsmokers.

3. Control high blood pressure. Follow your doctor's advice if you have high blood pressure.

4. Exercise regularly. Exercise increases the strength of your heart and improves circulation.

The Legs and Feet

1. Daily care of your feet can improve circulation and prevent infec-tions. See "Time Out for Footcare" for instructions on how to care for your feet.

2. If you have corns, callouses, or ingrown toenails, see a podiatrist (foot doctor). Tell him/her that you have diabetes. Avoid home reme-dies or "bathroom surgery."

Damage to the nerves may affect your ability to feel pain or tempera-ture. You may not be able to feel if your feet or legs are burned. They can burn from a heating pad, hot water bottle, or hot bath water. Avoid going barefoot. You may cut your foot and not feel it. See your doctor for any cuts or bruises on your feet. They could be very serious if healing is delayed.

Staying healthy with diabetes is a joint effort between you and your health team (doctor, nurse, dietitian, and pharmacist). Discuss with them any questions or concerns you have about your diabetes. Diabetes control depends on you. *Respect your complex and wonderful body!*

TIME OUT FOR FOOT CARE

Guidelines to Good Foot Care

1. Using warm water, never hot, wash feet daily and dry well.
2. Inspect feet carefully each day for open sores or irritation.
3. Apply lotion to feet to reduce dryness.
4. Trim nails every two weeks, straight across and even with end of toe.
5. Protect the feet from accidents by wearing comfortable, supportive shoes.
6. Avoid stockings that leave indentations under the elastic tops.
7. Avoid hot water and heating pads due to the risk of burns.

8. Avoid the use of commercial products to remove corns or callouses; consult a physician or podiatrist.

9. Consult your doctor if a sore or irritation does not heal promptly.

The Buerger-Allen Exercises

These exercises are designed:

- To increase foot comfort
- To improve blood flow to and from the feet
- Encouraged for all people concerned with the health of their feet
- To be done twice daily.

1. Lie on the bed with legs elevated for 3 minutes.

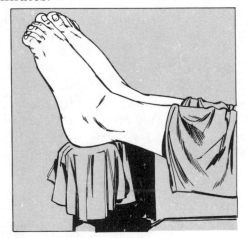

2. Sit on the side of the bed or chair, straighten knees, and lift heels off floor.

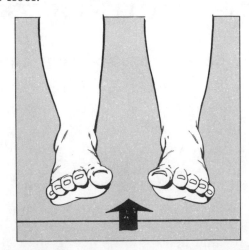

3. Point toes toward the floor.

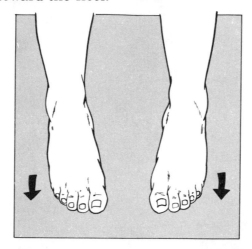

4. Point toes toward the ceiling.

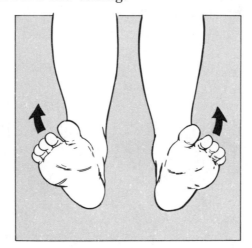

5. Point toes inward as far as possible.

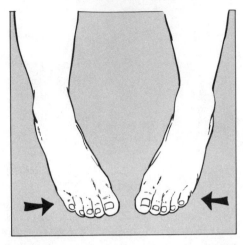

6. Point toes outward as far as possible.

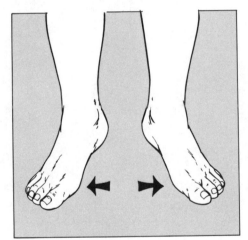

7. Point toes toward the ceiling, this time spreading toes.

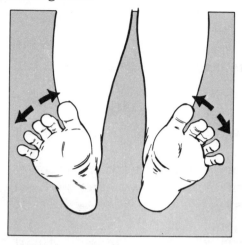

8. Point toes toward the floor, this time curling toes tightly.

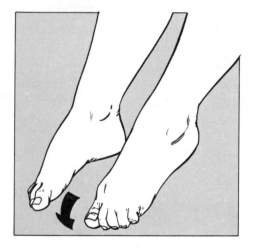

Evaluate Yourself 1

1. Because diabetes affects circulation and nerves, what parts of the body need special care?

2. How should you care for your:

   eyes?

   teeth?

   heart?

kidneys?

feet?

3. What are the Buerger-Allen exercises?

Answers to Evaluate Yourself 1

1. The eyes, mouth, kidneys, heart, feet, and legs need special care in diabetics.

2. **eyes:** Visit an ophthalmologist once per year, and control your blood sugar.

   teeth: Visit your dentist twice a year and control your blood sugar. Floss and brush your teeth. If you wear dentures, check your mouth daily for sores.

   heart: Follow your diet. Achieve your ideal body weight. Avoid smoking and control high blood pressure. Get regular exercise and control your blood sugar.

   kidneys: Drink 8 cups of fluids per day. Promptly report signs of a bladder infection. Control your blood sugar.

   feet: Wash feet daily. Avoid going barefoot. Do not use hot water bottles or heating pads. Do a daily inspection of your feet and avoid "bathroom" surgery.

3. The Buerger-Allen exercises are for the feet and legs, to be done twice daily. Increase foot comfort. Improve blood flow to and from the feet.

III

RECIPES

POINTS OF INTEREST

This part of *Diabetes: Recipes for Health* contains recipes that you can use from morning until night.

Each recipe here contains the:

- exchanges in one serving
- carbohydrate, protein, and fat content in grams
- sodium and potassium content in milligrams

When the nutrient content of a serving is transferred into exchanges, the number of grams of carbohydrate, protein, or fat may not exactly equal the nutrient content of an exchange.

For instance, a serving of Tomato Aspic Salad contains 5 grams of protein and 6 grams of carbohydrate. A vegetable serving comes closest to these two numbers. A vegetable serving contains 2 grams of protein and 5 grams of carbohydrate. There are some extra grams of protein and carbohydrate. But that is okay. It is close enough.

In other recipes, the exchanges do not seem to match the ingredients. For instance, 1 serving of Pumpkin Custard is 1 vegetable exchange and ½ meat, medium-fat exchange. And yet, this recipe does not include any fruit exchanges.

This is due to the fact that the number of grams of carbohydrate in one servng is about the same amount found in one fruit exchange.

One serving of Pumpkin Custard contains 7 grams of carbohydrate. And one fruit exchange contains 10 grams of carbohydrate.

Keep in mind that if you substitute some of the ingredients, you will be changing the sodium content of one serving. If the recipe calls for frozen peas and you use canned peas, you will be eating extra sodium.

Some other recipes are free foods. These contain twenty or fewer calories per serving.

There are some recipes that contain sugar, not a sugar substitute. During the holiday season, from Thanksgiving through New Years, you may prepare or eat special dessert foods.

When you eat a small portion, the serving does not contain a large amount of sugar. The sugar content is counted as part of your carbohydrate source.

Plan ahead. Make wise food choices. Eat and drink small servings. Keep in mind, your special treats are not a substitute for a balanced, nutritious meal.

APPETIZERS

Dips, Sauces, Dressings, Jam, and Jelly

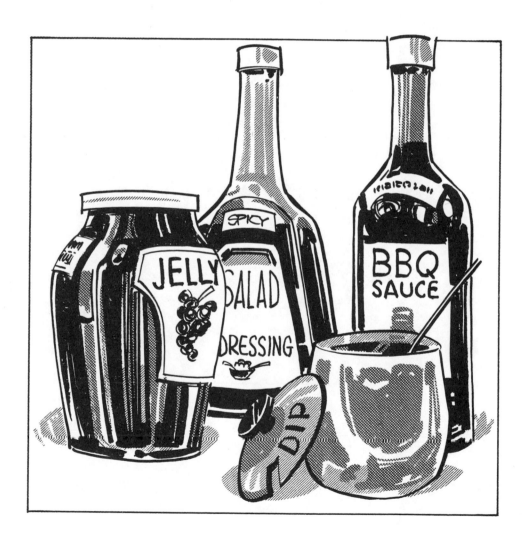

Bacon Tater Bites

50 tater tots
25 slices bacon
20 slices American cheese

1. Cook half-slices of bacon until brown but still limp.

2. Prepare tater tots according to package directions.

3. Cut slices of cheese in thirds and wrap a strip of cheese around each tater tot.

4. Wrap bacon around cheese and secure with toothpick.

Yield: 50 appetizers
3 appetizers: 1 vegetable exchange
             1 meat, medium fat exchange
             2 fat exchanges

Protein	9 gm
Fat	15 gm
Carbohydrate	4 gm
Sodium	210 mg
Potassium	87 mg
Calories	187

Olive Cheese Balls

½ cup butter, melted
2 cups sharp cheddar cheese, grated
1 cup flour
48 green olives, stuffed

1. Mix first three ingredients.

2. Flatten cheese mixture out.

3. Use a glass or cutter, 3 inches in diameter, to cut cheese wrap for olives. Wrap around olives.

4. Refrigerate overnight or freeze.

5. Bake at 450 degrees for 8–10 minutes.

Yield: 48 cheese balls

3 cheese balls: ½ fruit exchange		
1½ fat exchanges	Protein	4 gm
	Fat	12 gm
OR	Carbohydrate	6 gm
	Sodium	384 mg
½ milk exchange	Potassium	27 mg
1 fat exchange	Calories	148

Bread and Butter Pickles

4 cups cucumber, ⅛ inch slices
1 cup onion, ⅛ inch slices
1 garlic clove
2 tbsp salt, medium coarse
14–18 ice cubes
1 cup cider vinegar
1 cup water
1¼ tsp mustard seed
¾ tsp celery seed
½ tsp tumeric
3½–4 tsp liquid artificial sweetener

1. Combine cucumber, onion, and garlic in large bowl. Sprinkle with salt. Cover with ice cubes. Let stand overnight.

2. Drain well.

3. Combine remaining ingredients except liquid artificial sweetener in a 4-quart pan.

4. Add cucumber mixture. Bring to a boil. Cover and boil gently for two minutes.

5. Stir in liquid artificial sweetener.

6. Remove garlic clove.

7. Spoon into sterile jars. Seal.

Yield: 5 cups
½ cup: 1 vegetable exchange

Protein	1 gm
Fat	0 gm
Carbohydrate	6 gm
Sodium	1287 mg
Potassium	221 mg
Calories	28

Tailgate Chinese Chicken

3 lbs chicken wings
⅓ cup soy sauce
3 tbsp vinegar
3 tbsp granulated sugar
3 tbsp brown sugar
1 tsp ground ginger
2 cloves garlic, crushed

1. Disjoint chicken wings and discard tip ends.

2. Stir together soy sauce, vinegar, sugars, ginger, and garlic for marinade.

3. Put wings in heavy plastic bag and pour in marinade.

4. Close bag and place in a bowl, in case the bag leaks.

5. Marinate at least 2 hours, over night is best.

6. To cook, place in a 13 x 9 inch oblong pan and bake 350 degrees for over 1 hour.

Yield: 12 servings

1 serving: ½ bread-starch exchange 2 meat, low-fat exchanges		
Protein	17 gm
Fat	7 gm
Carbohydrate	8 gm
Sodium	571 mg
Potassium	43 mg
Calories	163

Deviled Eggs

1 hard cooked egg
1½ tsp vinegar
⅛ tsp dry mustard
⅛ tsp salt
pepper to taste
paprika to garnish

1. Cut hard cooked egg in half lengthwise. Remove yolk.

2. Crush yolk and mix with vinegar, mustard, salt, and pepper.

3. Refill whites with egg yolk mixture and garnish with paprika.

Yield: 1 serving
1 egg: 1 meat, medium fat
       exchange

Protein	6 gm
Fat	6 gm
Carbohydrate	0 gm
Sodium	327 mg
Potassium	70 mg
Calories	78

Tangy Cocktail Sauce

½ cup unsweetened tomato sauce
1 tsp parsley, finely chopped
1 tsp horseradish
1 tsp lemon juice
½ tsp salt
½ tsp worcestershire sauce
¼ tsp liquid artificial sweetener

1. Combine above ingredients.

2. Chill.

3. Serve with seafood.

Yield: ½ cup
2 tbsp or less: free food exchange

Protein	0 gm
Fat	0 gm
Carbohydrate	2 gm
Sodium	434 mg
Potassium	130 mg
Calories	8

Shrimp Quiche Hors D'oeurves

1 package (8 oz) refrigerated butterflake dinner rolls
about 4 oz small cooked shrimp
1 egg
½ cup half and half
2 tbsp finely minced green onion
½ tsp salt
¼ tsp dill weed
⅛ tsp cayenne
½ cup (4 oz) shredded Swiss cheese

1. Generously grease 2 dozen 1¾ inch muffin cups.

2. Separate rolls into 24 equal pieces and press each piece into bottom and sides of muffin cup.

3. Divide shrimp evenly among pastry shells.

4. Beat together egg, cream, onion, salt, dill, and cayenne until well-blended.

5. Put 2 tsp of above mixture in each cup.

6. Sprinkle cheese over top.

7. Bake uncovered at 375 degrees for 20 minutes.

8. Cook 5 minutes.

9. Option: Remove from muffin pans and cool completely on racks. Package airtight and freeze. To reheat, place frozen quiches on a baking sheet. Bake at 375 degrees for 15 minutes.

Yield: 24

1 serving: ½ meat, medium-fat exchange ½ fruit exchange		
Protein	4 gm
Fat	3 gm
Carbohydrate	5 gm
Sodium	151 mg
Potassium	29 mg
Calories	63

OR

1 vegetable exchange
½ fat exchange

2 servings: 1 fruit exchange
1 meat, medium fat exchange

Protein	7 gm
Fat	6 gm
Carbohydrate	10 gm
Sodium	302 mg
Potassium	58 mg
Calories	122

Mexican Dip

2 lbs Velveeta cheese
2 whole tomatoes
¼ cup onion, chopped
½ cup milk
1 small can taco sauce
½ tsp salt
pinch of oregano
1 tsp green chili pepper
2 tsp oil

1. Saute onion and tomato in oil.

3. Melt cheese with milk.

3. Add onions, tomato, and spices to cheese mixture.

4. Serve hot in fondue pot. Add jalapeño pepper and/or juice to make dip spicy.

Yield: 6 cups

¼ cup:	½ vegetable exchange 1 meat, medium fat exchange 2 fat exchanges	Protein Fat Carbohydrate Sodium Potassium Calories	9 gm 17 gm 2 gm 497 mg 80 mg 197
⅓ cup:	½ vegetable exchange 1½ meat, medium fat exchanges 2 fat exchanges	Protein Fat Carbohydrate Sodium Potassium Calories	12 gm 16 gm 3 gm 663 mg 107 mg 204
½ cup:	1 vegetable exchange 2 meat, medium fat exchanges 3 fat exchanges	Protein Fat Carbohydrate Sodium Potassium Calories	18 gm 24 gm 4 gm 995 mg 161 mg 304

Cottage Cheese Dip

1 cup cottage cheese
1 thin slice of onion
1 strip green pepper
¼ tsp garlic salt
2 tbsp lemon juice
¼ tsp celery salt
pepper to season
1 tsp worcestershire sauce
dash of tabasco

1. Blend all ingredients for 6–10 seconds.

Yield: 2 cups
2 tbsp or less: free food
    exchange

1 tbsp:		
	Protein	1 gm
	Fat	0 gm
	Carbohydrate	0.5 gm
	Sodium	44 mg
	Potassium	9 mg
	Calories	6

5 tbsp: ½ meat, medium fat exchange		
	Protein	5 gm
	Fat	0 gm
	Carbohydrate	2.5 gm
	Sodium	220 mg
	Potassium	45 mg
	Calories	30

8 tbsp: 1 meat, medium fat exchange ½ fruit exchange Add 1 fat exchange to meal plan		
	Protein	8 gm
	Fat	0 gm
	Carbohydrate	4 gm
	Sodium	352 mg
	Potassium	72 mg
	Calories	48

Chipped Beef Dip

½ cup sour cream
2½ oz chipped beef
8 oz cream cheese
2 tbsp milk
½ cup green pepper, chopped
½ tsp garlic salt
¼ tsp pepper
2 tbsp butter
½ cup slivered almonds

---

1. Mix all ingredients except almonds and butter. Spread in pie tin.

2. Melt butter. Add almonds. Sprinkle over mixture.

3. Bake 15–20 minutes at 350 degrees.

Yield: 2 cups
1 tbsp: 1 fat exchange

Protein	1 gm
Fat	5 gm
Carbohydrate	1 gm
Sodium	61 mg
Potassium	31 mg
Calories	53

California Dip

2 cups cottage cheese
4 tsp lemon juice
1 envelope (1⅓ oz) dehydrated onion soup

1. Combine all ingredients in blender until creamy.

2. Serve with fresh vegetables, chips, or crackers.

Yield: 1 pint (2 cups)
2 tbsp: ½ meat, medium fat
   exchange

Protein	4 gm
Fat	2 gm
Carbohydrate	2 gm
Sodium	244 mg
Potassium	40 mg
Calories	43

Quick California Dip

1⅓ oz dehydrated onion soup mix
1 pint sour cream

1. Blend dehydrated onion soup mix with sour cream.

2. Chill.

Yield: 2 cups
2 tablespoons: 1 fat exchange

Protein	1 gm
Fat	6 gm
Carbohydrate	2 gm
Sodium	192 mg
Potassium	52 mg
Calories	66

Dill Dip

1 cup sour cream
1 cup "real" mayonnaise
1 tbsp dill
1 tsp garlic salt
1 tsp salt

1. Mix all ingredients.

2. Refrigerate for 24 hours.

Yield: 2 cups

1 tbsp: 1 fat exchange		
Protein	0 gm
Fat	7 gm
Carbohydrate	0 gm
Sodium	119 mg
Potassium	11 mg
Calories	63

2 tbsp: 3 fat exchanges		
Protein	0 gm
Fat	14 gm
Carbohydrate	0 gm
Sodium	238 mg
Potassium	22 mg
Calories	126

¼ cup: 5½ fat exchanges		
Protein	0 gm
Fat	28 gm
Carbohydrate	0 gm
Sodium	476 mg
Potassium	44 mg
Calories	252

Nippy Cheese Sauce

1 cup medium cream sauce
1 cup sharp cheddar cheese, shredded
¼ tsp worchestershire sauce
dry mustard to taste

1. To increase sauce, add 1 cup shredded sharp cheddar cheese, grated.

2. Stir until melted and smooth.

3. Add dry mustard and worcestershire sauce.

Yield: 1 cup

½ cup serving:
   3 meat, high fat exchanges
   1 bread-starch exchange
   2 fat exchanges

Protein	19 gm
Fat	30 gm
Carbohydrate	13 gm
Sodium	913 mg
Potassium	233 mg
Calories	398

⅓ cup serving:
   2 meat, high fat exchanges
   ⅔ bread-starch exchange
   1 fat exchange

Protein	13 gm
Fat	19 gm
Carbohydrate	9 gm
Sodium	608 mg
Potassium	155 mg
Calories	259

Cream Sauce—Medium

2 tbsp margarine
2 tbsp flour
¼ tsp salt
1 cup skim milk

1. Melt margarine.

2. Add flour, salt, and a little of the milk to make a smooth paste. Gradually add rest of the milk.

3. Cook slowly, stirring constantly, until thickened over a slow heat in double boiler or very heavy pot.

4. Add pepper if you wish.

Yield: 1 cup

⅓ cup:	½ bread-starch exchange	Protein	3 gm
	1½ fat exchanges	Fat	7 gm
		Carbohydrate	8 gm
		Sodium	311 mg
		Potassium	124 mg
		Calories	107

½ cup:	½ meat, medium fat exchange	Protein	5 gm
	1½ fat exchanges	Fat	11 gm
	¾ bread starch exchange	Carbohydrate	12 gm
		Sodium	467 mg
		Potassium	186 mg
		Calories	167

Note: Make sauce 1 quart at a time and use for many varied meals.

Cranberry Orange Relish

2 lbs cranberries
juice from 2 oranges

1. Clean and dry thoroughly 2 pounds of fresh cranberries.

2. Freeze overnight.

3. Grind cranberries without thawing.

4. Squeeze the juice from 2 oranges and then grind the rind.

5. Mix altogether with sugar substitute to taste.

Yield: 4 cups (48 tbsp)
1 tbsp: free food exchange

Protein	0 gm
Fat	0 gm
Carbohydrate	2 gm
Sodium	0 mg
Potassium	20 mg
Calories	8

Cranberry Relish

1 lb or 4-4½ cups cranberries, fresh
1 pulp and rind of an orange, fresh (save juice)
1 tbsp liquid artificial sweetener

1. Grind cranberries and orange.

2. Stir in liquid artificial sweetener and reserved orange juice.

3. Refrigerate at least 4 hours before serving.

Yield: 2 cups
1 serving: ⅛ cup or less—free food
            exchange (2 tbsp)
¼ cup: ½ fruit exchange

Protein	0 gm
Fat	0 gm
Carbohydrate	6 gm
Sodium	1 mg
Potassium	48 mg
Calories	24

Candied Cranberries

1-16 ounce package cranberries (4 cups)
2½ cups sugar

1. Spread the cranberries in the bottom of a greased 13x9x2 inch baking pan.

2. Sprinkle cranberries with sugar.

3. Let stand at room temperature for 30 minutes.

4. Stir.

5. Cover with foil and bake at 350 degrees for 45–50 minutes.

6. Stir the cranberries occasionally by carefully lifting and turning cranberries with a metal spatula.

7. Chill until ready to use.

Yield: 3 cups
1 tbsp: 1 fruit exchange

Protein	0 gm
Fat	0 gm
Carbohydrate	11 gm
Sodium	0 mg
Potassium	8 mg
Calories	44

Rhubarb Sauce

4 cups fresh rhubarb, cut
½ cup water
1 tbsp liquid artificial sweetener

1. Add water to rhubarb in pan.

2. Cook rhubarb covered until soft.

3. Cool.

4. Add liquid artificial sweetener.

5. A dash of nutmeg may be added after cooking, if desired.

Yield: 4 servings
1 serving: ½ fruit exchange

Protein	1 gm
Fat	0 gm
Carbohydrate	7 gm
Sodium	2 mg
Potassium	306 mg
Calories	32

Barbecue Sauce

1 cup water
½ cup catsup
¼ cup finely chopped dill pickle
½ tsp salt
½ tsp dry mustard
½ tsp liquid artificial sweetener
⅛ tsp chili powder
a few drops of tabasco sauce

1. Blend all ingredients well.

Yield: 1½ cups
1–3 tbsp: free food exchange
       1 tbsp:

Protein	0 gm
Fat	0 gm
Carbohydrate	1 gm
Sodium	164 mg
Potassium	26 mg
Calories	4

Low Calorie Cumberland Sauce

8 oz jar low calorie apple jelly
1 tbsp orange juice
1 tsp lemon juice
1 tsp orange rind
1 tsp lemon rind
½ tsp dry mustard
⅛ tsp salt
⅛ tsp ginger

1. Combine ingredients in saucepan.

2. Heat, stirring constantly, until jelly melts.

3. Cook until mixture is smooth.

4. Serve hot or cold with baked ham or poultry.

Yield: 1 cup
3 tbsp or less: free food exchange

1 tbsp:		
	Protein	0 gm
	Fat	0 gm
	Carbohydrate	1 gm
	Sodium	16 mg
	Potassium	10 mg
	Calories	4

5 tbsp: ½ fruit exchange		
	Protein	0 gm
	Fat	0 gm
	Carbohydrate	5 gm
	Sodium	90 mg
	Potassium	50 mg
	Calories	20

Zero Dressing

½ cup tomato juice
1 tbsp lemon juice or vinegar
1 tbsp onion, finely chopped
⅛ tsp salt
pepper to taste

1. Combine ingredients in a jar with a tightly fitted top.

2. Shake well before using.

3. Chopped parsley, green pepper, horseradish, or mustard may be added if desired. Take into account the sodium content of horseradish and mustard.

Yield: about ⅔ cup (10 tbsp)
1 tbsp: free food exchange

Protein	0 gm
Fat	0 gm
Carbohydrate	0.8 gm
Sodium	51 mg
Potassium	35 mg
Calories	3

Yogurt Dressing

1-8 ounce container plain, unflavored yogurt (1 cup)
2 tbsp salad oil
1 tbsp lemon juice
1 tsp paprika
1 tsp salt
¼ tsp garlic powder
dash of hot pepper sauce

1. In small bowl with wire whisk or fork, stir all ingredients until well mixed.

2. Cover and refrigerate to use within 1 week.

3. Stir well before using.

Yield: 1 cup (16 tablespoons)
2 tablespoons: 1 fat exchange

Protein	1 gm
Fat	4 gm
Carbohydrate	2 gm
Sodium	282 mg
Potassium	46 mg
Calories	48

Yogurt Thousand Island Dressing

2 tbsp chili sauce
2 tbsp pickle relish
1 tbsp finely chopped onion
1 tsp vinegar
1 tsp prepared mustard
½ tsp salt
1 cup plain yogurt

1. Blend together chili sauce, relish, onion, vinegar, mustard, and salt. Fold in yogurt.

2. Cover and chill.

Yield: 1¼ cups (20 tbsp.)

2 tbsp: free food exchange

Protein	1 gm
Fat	0 gm
Carbohydrate	3 gm
Sodium	176 mg
Potassium	48 mg
Calories	16

4 tbsp: ½ fruit exchange

Protein	2 gm
Fat	0 gm
Carbohydrate	6 gm
Sodium	332 mg
Potassium	96 mg
Calories	32

Dressing

1 cup creamed cottage cheese
½ cup buttermilk
1 tsp lemon juice
¼ tsp salt
add chopped chives, parsley, or other herbs before using

1. Combine all ingredients in blender until perfectly smooth.

2. Refrigerate at least one hour before using. (Does not stand up under heat, on soups or hot dishes, but is great on cold fruit and salads.)

Yield: 1½ cups

2 tbsp: free food exchange

Protein	3 gm
Fat	1 gm
Carbohydrate	1 gm
Sodium	100 mg
Potassium	30 mg
Calories	25

5 tbsp: 1 meat, low fat exchange

Protein	7 gm
Fat	2 gm
Carbohydrate	2.5 gm
Sodium	250 mg
Potassium	75 mg
Calories	56

Easy Sour Cream Dressing

1 cup cottage cheese
2 tsp lemon juice
4 tbsp skim milk

1. Combine cottage cheese and lemon juice in blender. Blend until creamy.

2. Add skim milk a tablespoon at a time to desired consistency.

Yield: 1 cup

2 tbsp: ½ meat, low-fat exchange		
Protein	4 gm
Fat	1 gm
Carbohydrate	1 gm
Sodium	66 mg
Potassium	36 mg
Calories	29

4 tbsp: 1 meat, low-fat exchange		
Protein	8 gm
Fat	2 gm
Carbohydrate	2 gm
Sodium	132 mg
Potassium	72 mg
Calories	68

Sour Cream Dressing

1 cup sour cream (20%) or plain yogurt
2 tbsp prepared mustard
1 tsp lemon juice
½ tsp onion salt
½ tsp salt
½ tsp liquid artificial sweetener

1. Mix well.

2. Serve with tossed green or a potato salad.

Yield: 1 cup
Sour Cream: 1 tbsp = ½ fat
        exchange
       2 tbsp = 1 fat
        exchange
       1 tbsp:

Protein	0 gm
Fat	3 gm
Carbohydrate	0.5 gm
Sodium	120 mg
Potassium	18 mg
Calories	27

Yogurt: 1–4 tbsp = free food
     exchange
    5 tbsp = 1 vegetable
     exchange
    1 tbsp:

Protein	0.5 gm
Fat	0 gm
Carbohydrate	0.8 gm
Sodium	122 mg
Potassium	22 mg
Calories	5

Apple Jelly

1 envelope or 1 tbsp unflavored gelatin
3 cups unsweetened apple juice
2 tbsp liquid artificial sweetener
2 tbsp lemon juice
3 drops yellow food coloring
3 drops red food coloring

1. Soften gelatin in ¼ cup apple juice.

2. Heat 2¾ cups apple juice with liquid artificial sweetener, lemon juice, and food coloring.

3. Stir in softened gelatin.

4. Bring to a boil.

5. Pour into sterilized half pint jars.

6. Cover tightly.

7. Refrigerate.

TIP: For a more "jelly-like" flavor, add ½ bottle (6–7 tbsp) fruit pectin. Boil 1 minute.

Yield: about 2 pints
1 serving: 3 tbsp or less—free food exchange
1 tbsp:

Protein	0 gm
Fat	0 gm
Carbohydrate	1.4 gm
Sodium	0 mg
Potassium	12 mg
Calories	22

7 tbsp: 1 fruit exchange

Protein	0 gm
Fat	0 gm
Carbohydrate	10 gm
Sodium	0 mg
Potassium	84 mg
Calories	40

Blueberry Jam

4 cups blueberries
1¾ oz package powdered fruit pectin
1 tbsp lemon juice
1 tbsp liquid artificial sweetener

1. Crush blueberries in 3-quart saucepan.

2. Stir in powdered fruit pectin and lemon juice.

3. Bring to a boil. Boil and stir about 10 minutes or until 2 drops of the mixture slides off the side of a spoon.

4. Remove from heat.

5. Stir in liquid artificial sweetener.

6. Pour into sterile jars. Seal.

Yield: 1⅔ cups
1 serving: 1 tbsp or less—free food
       exchange
     2 tbsp—½ fruit
       exchange

1 tbsp:		2 tbsp:	
Protein	0 gm	Protein	0 gm
Fat	0 gm	Fat	0 gm
Carbohydrate	3 gm	Carbohydrate	6 gm
Sodium	0 mg	Sodium	0 mg
Potassium	21 mg	Potassium	42 mg
Calories	12	Calories	24

SALADS

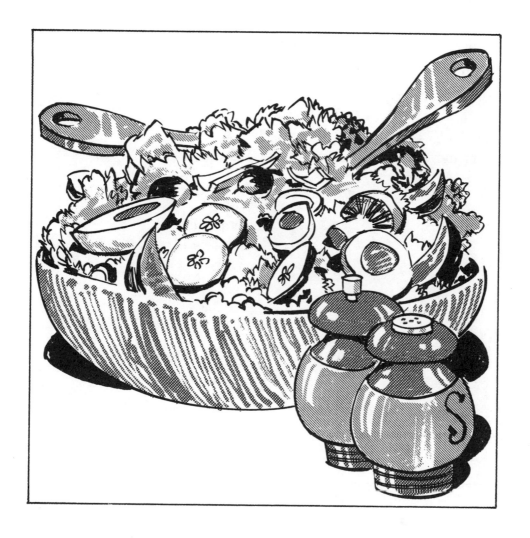

Molded Banana

1 small banana
½ envelope gelatin
½ cup boiling water
½ cup cold water

1. Dissolve gelatin in boiling water.

2. Add cold water and cool to room temperature.

3. Slice ½ banana into individual molds.

4. Pour gelatin over fruit and stir.

5. Chill until set.

Yield: 2 servings
1 serving: 1 fruit exchange

Protein	2 gm
Fat	0 gm
Carbohydrate	8 gm
Sodium	0 mg
Potassium	146 mg
Calories	40

Apple Cider Salad

2¼ tsp unflavored gelatin
2⅔ tbsp cold water
1 tsp liquid artificial sweetener
1 cup apple juice, unsweetened
1 tbsp lemon juice
¼ tsp salt
⅔ cup applesauce, unsweetened

1. Soften gelatin in cold water.

2. Combine liquid artificial sweetener, apple juice, lemon juice, and salt.

3. Heat and add the above to the softened gelatin stirring until gelatin dissolves.

4. Cool until mixture begins to thicken. Fold in applesauce. Chill until set in individual molds.

Yield: 4 servings
1 serving: 1 fruit exchange

Protein	2 gm
Fat	0 gm
Carbohydrate	12 gm
Sodium	134 mg
Potassium	99 mg
Calories	56

Cranberry Christmas Salad

1-1 lb can whole cranberry sauce
1-3 oz package red jello
1 cup boiling water
¼ tsp salt
1 tbsp lemon juice
½ cup mayonnaise salad dressing
1 medium apple diced and peeled
¼ cup chopped walnuts

1. Heat sauce and strain. Save juice. Set cranberries aside.

2. Dissolve jello in hot juice and water.

3. Add salt and lemon juice.

4. Chill until thick.

5. Beat in mayonnaise until light and fluffy.

6. Fold in cranberries, fruit, and nuts.

7. Pour in mold.

8. Chill until set.

Yield: 12 servings
1 serving: 2½ fruit exchanges
          ½ fat exchange

Protein	1 gm
Fat	3 gm
Carbohydrate	25 gm
Sodium	125 mg
Potassium	16 mg
Calories	131

Cranberry Salad (Molded)

½ cup raw cranberries
1 small apple, cored
½ whole orange
½ tsp liquid artificial sweetener
½ envelope cherry-flavored artificially sweetened gelatin
1 tsp lemon juice
½ cup boiling water

1. Dissolve gelatin in boiling water.

2. Grind cranberries, orange, and apple together.

3. Add liquid artificial sweetener and lemon juice.

4. When gelatin begins to set, stir in cranberry mixture and pour into square pan.

5. Chill until set. Serve on lettuce leaf.

Yield: 4 servings.
1 serving: ½ fruit exchange

Protein	0 gm
Fat	0 gm
Carbohydrate	7 gm
Sodium	1 mg
Potassium	90 mg
Calories	28

Grapefruit-Orange Mold

2 envelopes lemon-flavored artificially sweetened gelatin
¼ tsp salt
1 cup boiling water
¾ cup cold water
¾ cup fresh diced grapefruit sections
¾ cup fresh orange sections, drained

1. Dissolve gelatin and salt in boiling water.

2. Add water to gelatin mixture.

3. Chill until very thick.

4. Fold in grapefruit and orange sections.

5. Pour into six individual molds.

6. Chill until firm.

Yield: 6 servings
1 serving: ½ fruit exchange

Protein	0 gm
Fat	0 gm
Carbohydrate	5 gm
Sodium	89 mg
Potassium	79 mg
Calories	20

Melon-Grape Mold

1 envelope artificially sweetened gelatin
2 cups hot water
2 tbsp lemon juice
1 cup cantaloupe, diced
8 green grapes

1. Dissolve gelatin in hot water.

2. Cool.

3. Combine diced cantaloupe and grapes in individual molds.

4. Pour gelatin mixture into molds.

5. Allow to set overnight.

Yield: 2 servings
1 serving: 1 fruit exchange

Protein	0 gm
Fat	0 gm
Carbohydrate	10 gm
Sodium	10 mg
Potassium	256 mg
Calories	40

Spiced Peach Salad (Molded)

1 envelope orange-flavored artificially sweetened gelatin
1 cup water
4 whole cloves
⅛ tsp cinnamon, ground
1 tbsp vinegar
6 (1 can) unsweetened peach halves

1. Simmer cloves and cinnamon in water ½ hour.

2. Remove whole cloves.

3. Dissolve gelatin in the spiced water.

4. Allow to cool.

5. Add vinegar after mixture has cooled.

6. Slice one peach half into each of six individual molds.

7. Pour gelatin mixture into molds. Allow to set.

8. Unmold on lettuce leaf.

9. Garnish with a sprig of parsley.

Yield: 6 servings
1 serving: ½ fruit exchange

Protein	0 gm
Fat	0 gm
Carbohydrate	6 gm
Sodium	0 mg
Potassium	137 mg
Calories	24

Golden Pineapple Salad

2½ envelopes lemon-flavored artificially sweetened gelatin
1¼ cups cold water
1¼ cups hot water
⅔ cup unsweetened pineapple chunks, drained
1 large orange, diced
5 unsweetened bing cherries, pitted and drained

1. Dissolve gelatin in hot water.

2. Add cold water.

3. Let stand until mixture starts to gel.

4. Add drained pineapple and diced orange to gelatin. Stir.

5. When set, cut and place on lettuce leaf.

6. Garnish with unsweetened bing cherry.

Yield: 5 servings
1 serving: ½ fruit exchange

Protein	0 gm
Fat	0 gm
Carbohydrate	7 gm
Sodium	0 mg
Potassium	93 mg
Calories	28

Pineapple Lime Salad

½ cup unsweetened pineapple, canned and diced
1 tsp celery, diced
1 tsp pimento, chopped
1 tbsp vinegar
1 envelope lime-flavored artificially sweetened gelatin
½ cup hot water

1. Dissolve the gelatin in hot water.

2. When it begins to set, add the fruit, celery, and pimentos which have been marinated in the vinegar and salt.

3. Put into two individual molds and let stand until set.

4. Unmold and serve on crisp lettuce leaf.

Yield: 2 servings
1 serving: ½ fruit exchange

Protein	0 gm
Fat	0 gm
Carbohydrate	5 gm
Sodium	267 mg
Potassium	63 mg
Calories	20

Waldorf Salad (Jellied)

2 tbsp light or dark raisins
3 tbsp carrots, grated
¾ cup red apples, diced, unpared
3 tbsp walnuts, coarsely chopped
1½ envelopes lemon-flavored artificially sweetened gelatin
½ cup hot water
½ cup cold water

1. Let raisins stand in boiling water.

2. Drain.

3. Combine raisins, carrots, apples, and walnuts.

4. Divide equally into three individual molds.

5. Dissolve gelatin in hot water.

6. Add cold water.

7. Pour over mixture in the molds. Chill until firm.

8. Serve on crisp lettuce leaf.

Yield: 3 servings
1 serving: 1 fruit exchange
          1 fat exchange

Protein	1 gm
Fat	4 gm
Carbohydrate	11 gm
Sodium	4 mg
Potassium	139 mg
Calories	84

Perfection Salad

2 envelopes lime-flavored artificially sweetened gelatin
1¾ cups boiling water
3 tbsp vinegar
1½ tbsp lemon juice
1 cup shredded cabbage
2 tbsp minced pimento
1 cup diced celery
½ cup diced carrots
½ tsp liquid artificial sweetener

1. Pour boiling water over gelatin.

2. Stir until dissolved.

3. Add vinegar, lemon juice, and liquid artificial sweetener.

4. Chill until liquid starts to congeal. Then, add chopped vegetables.

5. Stir and pour into square pan.

6. Chill until firm.

7. Cut into squares.

8. Place on lettuce leaf.

Yield: 4 servings
1 serving: 1 vegetable exchange

Protein	3 gm
Fat	0 gm
Carbohydrate	5 gm
Sodium	51 mg
Potassium	240 mg
Calories	32

Golden Glow Salad

2½ envelopes orange-flavored artificially sweetened gelatin
2¼ cups boiling water
1½ tbsp vinegar
1½ tbsp lemon juice
½ cup shredded carrots
½ cup diced celery
½ tsp liquid artificial sweetener

1. Pour boiling water over gelatin and stir until dissolved.

2. Add vinegar and lemon juice and liquid artificial sweetener.

3. Chill.

4. When gelatin begins to congeal, add vegetables. Pour into square pan.

5. Place in refrigerator. Chill until firm.

6. Cut into squares; place on lettuce leaf.

Yield: 5 servings
1 serving: free food exchange

Protein	0 gm
Fat	0 gm
Carbohydrate	2 gm
Sodium	20 mg
Potassium	88 mg
Calories	4

Carrot Orange Mold

1 tbsp unflavored gelatin or orange-flavored artificially
  sweetened gelatin
½ cup orange juice
1 tsp liquid artificial sweetener
1 cup hot water
1 tbsp vinegar
¼ tsp salt
½ cup raw carrots, shredded
½ cup pineapple tidbits, unsweetened, drained
½ cup fresh orange sections, cubed, drained

1. Sprinkle gelatin on cold orange juice to soften.

2. Add softened gelatin to very hot water and stir until thoroughly
   dissolved.

3. Add salt, vinegar, and artificial sweetener.

4. Chill until thickened.

5. Fold in carrots, pineapple, and orange.

6. Turn into mold and chill until firm.

Yield: 6 servings
1 serving: ½ fruit exchange

Protein	1 gm
Fat	0 gm
Carbohydrate	7 gm
Sodium	94 mg
Potassium	124 mg
Calories	32

Fresh Vegetable Salad (Jellied)

3½ envelopes lime-flavored artificially sweetened gelatin
¾ tsp salt
1 cup hot water
¾ cup cold water
2 tbsp vinegar
½ cup diced cucumber
½ cup celery, chopped fine
¾ cup diced tomatoes

1. Dissolve gelatin and salt in hot water.

2. Add cold water and vinegar.

3. Chill until slightly thickened.

4. Combine vegetables and fold into gelatin mixture.

5. Pour into molds or serving pan. Chill until firm.

6. Serve on crisp lettuce.

Yield: 6 servings
1 serving: free food exchange

Protein	0 gm
Fat	0 gm
Carbohydrate	2 gm
Sodium	281 mg
Potassium	151 mg
Calories	8

Tomato Aspic Salad

1 cup tomato juice or V-8 juice
½ leaf bay leaf
2 tsp plain gelatin
½ cup celery, diced
2 tsp onion, chopped
¼ cup water, cold

1. Simmer tomato, bayleaf, celery, and onion.

2. Soak gelatin in cold water.

3. Drain and strain the boiling liquid from the vegetables which are cooking.

4. Pour this boiling liquid over the softened gelatin to dissolve it.

5. Pour into individual molds.

6. Set in a cold place until firm.

7. Serve on a lettuce leaf.

8. Garnish with parsley.

Yield: 2 servings
1 serving: 1 vegetable exchange

Protein	5 gm
Fat	0 gm
Carbohydrate	6 gm
Sodium	280 mg
Potassium	383 mg
Calories	44

Fresh Vegetable Relish

¾ **cup tomato, diced**
¼ **cup green pepper, diced**
¾ **cup cucumber, diced**
¼ **cup dill pickle, diced**
½ **cup Zero dressing**

1. Combine vegetables in pan and pour dressing over them.

2. Stir to combine vegetables and to cover with dressing.

3. Let stand in refrigerator for not more than two hours.

4. Drain dressing off before serving.

Yield: 4 servings
1 serving: 1 vegetable exchange

Protein	1 gm
Fat	0 gm
Carbohydrate	6 gm
Sodium	374 mg
Potassium	339 mg
Calories	28

Carrot Raisin Salad

⅓ **cup raw carrots, grated**
1 **tsp raisins**
1 **tsp mayonnaise**

1. Mix ingredients and place on lettuce leaf.

Yield: 1 serving
1 serving: 1 vegetable exchange
           ½ fat exchange

Protein	1 gm
Fat	2 gm
Carbohydrate	6 gm
Sodium	44 mg
Potassium	161 mg
Calories	46

Vegetable Salad Supreme

1 cup cooked peas
1 cup cooked diced carrots
1 cup cooked diced green beans
⅛ tsp celery salt
¼ tsp paprika
½ tsp salt
½ cup Zero dressing

1. Mix all ingredients and marinate in Zero dressing (covering the vegetables) for one hour.

2. Drain off excess liquid.

3. Serve on lettuce leaf.

4. Top with sprig of parsley.

Yield: 6 servings
1 serving: 1 vegetable exchange

Protein	2 gm
Fat	0 gm
Carbohydrate	7 gm
Sodium	265 mg
Potassium	190 mg
Calories	36

Stuffed Tomato Salad

1 tomato, peeled
1 rounded tbsp cottage cheese
1 tbsp green pepper, chopped

1. Dip tomato in boiling water for a few seconds.

2. Peel, core, and chill tomato.

3. Cut from top halfway down as to make wedges.

4. Chop green peppers and mix with cottage cheese.

5. Place mixture in tomato.

6. Place on lettuce leaf.

7. Chill and serve.

Yield: 1 serving
1 serving: 1 vegetable exchange

Protein	2 gm
Fat	1 gm
Carbohydrate	7 gm
Sodium	69 mg
Potassium	344 mg
Calories	45

Corraines Salad

1 head lettuce, torn
1 green pepper, sliced
1 chopped onion
1-10 oz package of frozen peas (cooked and drained)
1 cup grated cheddar cheese
1 lb bacon fried (drained) and crumbled
1 cup real mayonnaise

1. Layer lettuce, green pepper, onion, and peas.

2. Top with grated cheese and bacon bits.

3. Frost top with mayonnaise.

4. Cover and refrigerate.

5. To serve, toss salad.

Yield: 20 servings
1 serving: free vegetable exchange

free vegetable exchange	Protein	4 gm
½ meat, high fat exchange	Fat	26 gm
	Carbohydrate	3 gm
4 fat exchanges	Sodium	261 mg
	Potassium	109 mg
	Calories	262

Endive Salad

1 head endive
3 slices bacon
½ raw onion, sliced
3 potatoes, medium
¼ cup vinegar

1. Clean endive and remove green portion. Cut. Add onion.

2. Cut bacon into small pieces. Fry. Save bacon grease (3 tbsp).

3. Boil potato. Mash. Save potato water.

4. Mix bacon grease, bacon, potato water, and vinegar.

5. Pour over endive and mix.

Yield: 4 quarts
Serves: 16

1 cup: free vegetable exchange ½ fat exchange		
Protein	1 gm
Fat	3 gm
Carbohydrate	2 gm
Sodium	22 mg
Potassium	102 mg
Calories	39

Coleslaw

½ cup cabbage, slawed
1 tsp vinegar
¼ tsp liquid artificial sweetener
parsley to garnish
⅛ tsp salt
⅛ tsp pepper

Yield: 1 serving

1 serving: free food exchange		
Protein	0 gm
Fat	0 gm
Carbohydrate	2 gm
Sodium	273 mg
Potassium	85 mg
Calories	8

Cabbage Salad

2 cups cabbage, shredded
1 cup crushed pineapple, water or juice packed, drained
1 large apple or 2 small apples
½ cup salad dressing, mayonnaise
1 tsp vinegar
artificial sweetener (equal to 1 tsp sugar)

1. Shred or chop cabbage. Core apples but do not peel. Chop apples but not too fine. Add pineapple.

2. Mix salad dressing, vinegar, and some sweetener (to taste).

3. Add this to other ingredients just before serving—this tends to get watery if it stands too long.

4. Toss lightly and put in serving bowls.

Yield: 4 cups
½ cup: 1 vegetable exchange
       ½ fat exchange

Protein	1 gm
Fat	3 gm
Carbohydrate	8 gm
Sodium	47 mg
Potassium	99 mg
Calories	63

Hot Mashed Potato Salad

4 small potatoes
1 hard cooked egg
small amount of diced onion, raw
vinegar to taste
⅛ tsp salt
pepper to taste

1. Boil and season potatoes as for mashing.

2. Mash with hard cooked egg and onion, using vinegar for moisture instead of milk or water.

Yield: 4 servings (2 cups)
1 serving: ½ cup serving: 1 bread-starch exchange

Protein	3 gm
Fat	1 gm
Carbohydrate	15 gm
Sodium	85 mg
Potassium	385 mg
Calories	81

Potato Salad

1 hard cooked egg, diced
½ cup potato, cooked, diced
1 tsp mayonnaise
2 tbsp onion
2 tbsp celery
2 tbsp green pepper
⅛ tsp salt
pepper to taste

Yield: 1 serving
1 serving: 1 meat, medium fat exchange
1 bread-starch exchange
1 fat exchange

Protein	8 gm
Fat	9 gm
Carbohydrate	14 gm
Sodium	378 mg
Potassium	478 mg
Calories	169

German Potato Salad

3 slices bacon
2 tbsp flour
⅔ cup cider vinegar
1⅓ cup water
1 tbsp minced onion
1 tsp salt
dash of pepper
1 tsp liquid sweetener
2 tsp chopped pimento
6 cups sliced cooked potatoes

1. Fry bacon until crisp. Drain on paper.

2. Reserve 2 tbsp drippings.

3. Crumble bacon.

4. Slowly blend flour in drippings.

5. Stir in vinegar, water, and onion. Cook until mixture boils and thickens, stirring constantly.

6. Simmer 10 minutes.

7. Stir in salt, pepper, liquid sweetener, and pimento.

8. Layer potatoes, bacon, and sauce in bowl.

9. Allow to stand for several hours.

10. Heat just before serving. Serve immediately.

Yield: 8 servings
1 serving: 1½ bread-starch
      exchanges

Protein	3 gm
Fat	1 gm
Carbohydrate	22 gm
Sodium	299 mg
Potassium	486 mg
Calories	109

24 Hour Fruit Salad

2 cups pineapple, water or juice pack, drained
4 oz cherries
1 cup miniature marshmallows
2 egg yolks
1 tbsp sugar
juice of one lemon
½ pint whipping cream

1. Boil egg yolks, sugar, and lemon juice until thick. Cool.

2. Add cream to egg mixture.

3. Add fruit, cherries, and marshmallows.

4. Refrigerate.

Yield: 1 quart

½ cup: 1½ fruit exchanges 1½ fat exchanges		
	Protein	2 gm
	Fat	7 gm
	Carbohydrate	15 gm
	Sodium	17 mg
	Potassium	117 mg
	Calories	131

¼ cup: 1 fruit exchange ½ fat exchange		
	Protein	1 gm
	Fat	3.5 gm
	Carbohydrate	7 gm
	Sodium	8 mg
	Potassium	58 mg
	Calories	63

Four Fruit Salad

¼ peach, unsweetened
¼ pear, unsweetened
½ of one ring of pineapple, unsweetened
3 cherries, unsweetened
¼ cup cottage cheese

1. Arrange fruit on crisp salad greens.

2. Top with ¼ cup of cottage cheese.

Yield: 1 serving
1 serving: 1 meat, low-fat
          exchange
      1 fruit exchange

Protein	8 gm
Fat	2 gm
Carbohydrate	10 gm
Sodium	129 mg
Potassium	207 mg
Calories	90

Pineapple Cottage Cheese Salad

1 unsweetened pineapple ring (⅜ inch)
¼ cup cottage cheese
lettuce leaf

1. Round cottage cheese on top of pineapple ring.

2. Serve on lettuce leaf.

Yield: 1 serving
1 serving: 1 meat, low fat
          exchange
      ½ fruit exchange

Protein	8 gm
Fat	2 gm
Carbohydrate	7 gm
Sodium	129 mg
Potassium	109 mg
Calories	78

Tangy Cottage Cheese Salad

½ envelope lime-flavored artificially sweetened gelatin
6 tbsp water
¾ cup cottage cheese
¼ cup shaved carrots
2 tbsp green pepper, chopped fine
½ tsp horseradish
¼ tsp salt
⅛ tsp liquid artificial sweetener
2 tbsp skim milk powder
2 tbsp cold water

1. Sprinkle gelatin over water in saucepan.

2. Cook over low heat.

3. Stir until dissolved.

4. Remove from heat.

5. Stir in cottage cheese, carrots, green pepper, horseradish, salt, and liquid artificial sweetener.

6. Beat skim milk powder and cold water until thick.

7. Fold into gelatin mixture.

8. Turn into individual molds.

9. Chill.

Yield: 4 servings

1 serving:	1 meat, low-fat exchange		Protein	7 gm
	½ fruit exchange		Fat	2 gm
			Carbohydrate	4 gm
	OR		Sodium	253 mg
			Potassium	136 mg
	½ meat, low-fat exchange		Calories	62
	1 vegetable exchange			

Tuna Salad

½ cup canned tuna
½ cup cooked macaroni
1 tbsp celery, diced
1 tsp mayonnaise
1 tsp minced pimento
⅛ tsp salt
pepper to taste

1. Toss ingredients together lightly with a fork.

2. Place in a lettuce cup and garnish with ½ hard cooked egg.

3. Chill.

Tuna may be substituted with 2 ounces diced, cooked chicken, ham, etc.

Yield: 1 serving

1 serving:	2 meat, low-fat exchanges 1½ bread-starch exchanges		
	Protein	19 gm
	Fat	5 gm
	Carbohydrate	21 gm
	Sodium	1108 mg
	Potassium	341 mg
	Calories	205

Tuna-Egg Salad

7 oz can water-packed tuna
1 hard cooked egg, diced
1 tbsp celery, diced
4 tsp mayonnaise (expand with small amount of milk)

1. Mix all ingredients well.

2. Serve on lettuce leaf with tomato wedges or serve as sandwich filling.

Yield: 4 servings

1 serving: 2 meat, low-fat exchanges	Protein	14 gm
	Fat	6 gm
1 sandwich: 2 meat, low-fat exchanges	Carbohydrate	0 gm
	Sodium	448 mg
2 bread-starch exchanges	Potassium	154 mg
	Calories	110

Egg Salad

1 hard cooked egg
1½ tsp vinegar
⅛ tsp dry mustard
⅛ tsp salt
pepper to taste
paprika to garnish

1. Mash and mix the entire egg with seasonings.

2. Serve as a salad on a lettuce leaf with tomato wedges or serve as filling for a sandwich.

Yield: 1 serving

Salad: 1 meat, medium-fat exchange	Protein	6 gm
	Fat	6 gm
Sandwich: 1 meat, medium-fat exchange	Carbohydrate	0 gm
	Sodium	327 mg
2 bread-starch exchanges	Potassium	70 mg
	Calories	78

Salmon and Cucumber Salad

2 cups diced cucumber
1 cup sliced celery
1 tsp Accent
12 oz canned salmon (well drained)
2 tsp mayonnaise (thinned with 1 tbsp vinegar)

1. Combine cucumber and celery.

2. Sprinkle with Accent.

3. Toss well to mix. Let stand while preparing remaining ingredients.

4. Flake salmon.

5. Combine with cucumber mixture and mayonnaise.

Yield: 6 servings

1 serving: 2 meat, medium fat exchanges		
1 vegetable exchange	Protein	16 gm
	Fat	10 gm
	Carbohydrate	4 gm
OR	Sodium	395 mg
	Potassium	220 mg
2 meat, low-fat exchanges	Calories	170
1 fat exchange		
1 vegetable exchange		

Turkey Salad Roll

2 oz turkey, cooked, diced
1 tbsp celery, diced
2 tbsp cream, sour cultured half and half
⅛ tsp salt
⅛ tsp pepper
1 small frankfurter roll
1 leaf of lettuce

1. Mix celery and turkey in bowl.

2. Add sour cream and toss.

3. Season with salt, pepper, and chill.

4. Split the roll lengthwise.

5. Place a lettuce leaf on each roll and fill with salad.

Yield: 1 serving

1 serving:		
2 meat, low-fat exchanges	Protein	21 gm
	Fat	12 gm
2 bread-starch exchanges	Carbohydrate	31 gm
	Sodium	617 mg
1 fat exchange	Potassium	337 mg
	Calories	316

BREADS

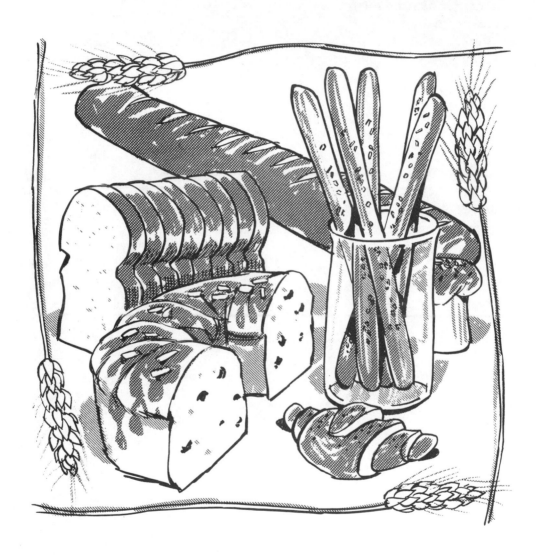

Diet Rolls

Pam Spray
3 eggs, separated
¼ tsp cream of tartar
3 tbsp cottage cheese
2 tsp sugar substitute

1. Preheat oven to 300 degrees. Spray cookie sheet with Pam.

2. Separate eggs very carefully, no yolk in whites.

3. Beat egg whites with cream of tartar until whites are stiff but not dry.

4. Fold in yolks, cottage cheese, and sugar substitute. Mix for no more than one minute.

5. Place mixture carefully on sheet, gently putting one tbsp on top of another until each roll is about 2 inches high. Repeat until you have six piles.

6. Place sheet in oven and bake one hour at 300 degrees.

Yield: 6 rolls
2 rolls: 1 meat, medium fat
       exchange

Protein	8 gm
Fat	6 gm
Carbohydrate	0 gm
Sodium	60 mg
Potassium	45 mg
Calories	86

Blueberry Muffins

1½ cups all-purpose flour
3 tsp baking powder
½ tsp salt
1 egg, well beaten
1 tsp liquid sweetener
½ cup skim milk
3 tbsp margarine (melted) or 3 tbsp corn oil
⅔ cup blueberries, fresh, frozen, well-drained or canned

1. Preheat oven to 400 degrees.

2. Mix together sifted flour, baking powder, and salt.

3. Add and blend well-beaten egg, milk, and liquid sweetener.

4. When partly blended, add melted margarine *or* oil. Blend just enough to combine the ingredients.

5. Fold in the blueberries.

6. Place paper muffin cups in muffin pan or on a cookie sheet.

7. Fill each cup ½ to ⅔ full.

8. Bake 25 minutes or until done at 350 degrees.

Yield: 12 muffins
1 muffin: 1 bread-starch exchange
        1 fat exchange

Protein	3 gm
Fat	4 gm
Carbohydrate	14 gm
Sodium	248 mg
Potassium	44 mg
Calories	104

Apple Cinnamon Coffee Cake

¼ cup soft shortening
½ cup sugar
1 egg
½ cup skim milk
1½ cups sifted flour
2 tsp baking powder
½ tsp salt
2 fresh apples, sliced, 2½ inch
1 tsp cinnamon
1 tsp sugar substitute

1. Cream shortening and sugar.

2. Beat in egg.

3. Add milk.

4. Sift together dry ingredients and blend into liquid mixture.

5. Spread batter in greased 9-inch square pan.

6. Arrange apple slices on top of batter, pressing them slightly into the batter.

7. Combine sugar substitute and cinnamon; sprinkle on top.

8. Bake at 375 degrees for 25 to 35 minutes.

Yield: 16-2¼ inch squares

Exchange: (2¼ inch squares)		
1 bread-starch	Protein	2 gm
exchange	Fat	4 gm
1 fat exchange	Carbohydrate	23 gm
1 fruit exchange	Sodium	110 mg
	Potassium	40 mg
	Calories	136

OR

Yield: 9-3x3 inch squares

Exchange: (1 3x3 inch square)		
2 bread-starch	Protein	3 gm
exchanges	Fat	7 gm
1 fruit exchange	Carbohydrate	41 gm
1½ fat exchanges	Sodium	197 mg
	Potassium	71 mg
	Calories	239

Apple Bread

1 cup margarine
2 cups sugar
4 eggs
4 cups flour
1 tsp salt
1 tsp vanilla
2 tsp baking soda
4 tbsp sour milk
4 cups apples, cut up
1 cup nuts, ground

Topping

4 tbsp flour
4 tbsp sugar
4 tbsp margarine
2 tsp cinnamon

1. Mix baking soda in milk.

2. Mix all ingredients.

3. Pour into four 8½ x 4½ inch pans.

4. Sprinkle topping over dough.

5. Bake 45 minutes at 370 degrees.

Yield: 72 one-half inch slices
1 serving: 2 fruit exchanges
            1 fat exchange

Protein	1 gm
Fat	5 gm
Carbohydrate	19 gm
Sodium	78 mg
Potassium	75 mg
Calories	125

Zucchini Bread

3 eggs
2 cups sugar
1 cup oil
2 cups zucchini, grated
3 cups flour
1 tsp baking powder
½ tsp baking soda
3 tsp cinnamon
1 cup nuts, ground

1. Beat eggs until foamy.

2. Mix in sugar, oil, and zucchini.

3. Add remaining ingredients.

4. Pour into bread pan.

5. Bake at 350 degrees for one hour.

6. Remove from pan immediately.

Yield: 36 one-quarter inch slices
1 serving: 1 bread-starch
                exchange
           1 fat exchange
           ½ fruit exchange

Protein	3 gm
Fat	10 gm
Carbohydrate	21 gm
Sodium	14 mg
Potassium	47 mg
Calories	186

Potato Lefse

4 cups boiled and riced potato (packed)
⅓ cup shortening
1 tbsp sugar
1¼ tsp salt
¼ cup milk, 2% fat
1½ cup flour

1. Mix first 5 ingredients together when warm. Cool.

2. Add flour.

3. Make into balls and roll thin on floured board.

4. Bake on ungreased griddle at 400 degrees. When bubbles show, turn. Cook until Lefse is brown. To store, place in folded towel. When cool, wrap in Gladwrap to keep soft. Freeze.

Yield: 24
1 serving: ⅔ bread-starch
exchange
½ fat exchange

Protein	2 gm
Fat	3 gm
Calories	11 gm
Sodium	144 mg
Potassium	114 mg
Calories	79

VEGETABLE DISHES

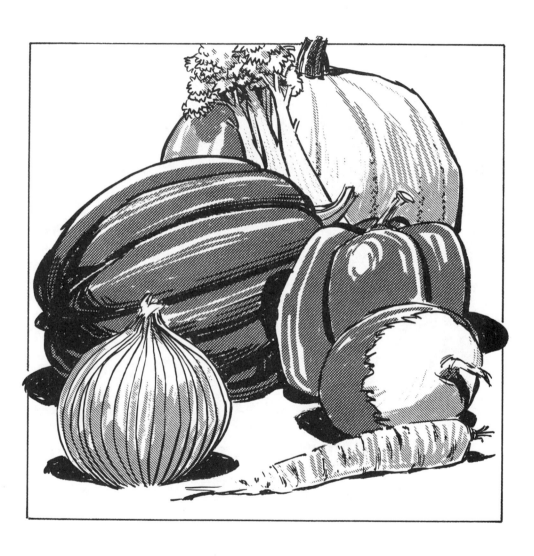

Sweet and Sour Beans

1 cup yellow wax beans
1 cup green beans
2 cups of liquid from beans
1 tbsp chopped onion
¾ tsp liquid artificial sweetener
2 tbsp vinegar
garnish with paprika
¼ tsp salt
¼ tsp pepper

1. Marinate beans in liquid, onion, liquid artificial sweetener, and vinegar for 2–3 hours or overnight.

2. Serve drained on lettuce in salad bowl.

3. Garnish with paprika.

Yield: 4 servings
1 serving: 1 vegetable exchange

Protein	1 gm
Fat	0 gm
Carbohydrate	4 gm
Sodium	134 mg
Potassium	113 mg
Calories	20

Wild Rice Casserole

1 cup wild rice
¼ cup white rice
½ cup celery, chopped
½ cup onion, chopped
1 green pepper, chopped
⅓ lb pork sausage
1 can cream of mushroom soup
1 can cream of chicken soup

1. Boil wild rice in water for 1 hour. Change water 2 times. Omit salt.

2. Boil white rice separately from wild rice.

3. Saute celery, onion, and green pepper.

4. Fry sausage. Drain off fat.

5. Mix all ingredients. Add cream soups.

6. Bake at 350 degrees until rice is done.

Yield: 2 quarts (16 servings)

½ cup: 1 bread-starch exchange 1 fat exchange		
Protein	3 gm
Fat	7 gm
Carbohydrate	16 gm
Sodium	375 mg
Potassium	98 mg
Calories	139

Pickled Beets

1-2 lb can whole beets (32 oz)
2 tbsp vinegar
6–8 cloves
⅓ tsp liquid sweetener

1. Boil all ingredients. Cool.

2. Color is improved by adding several drops of red food coloring.

Yield: 4 cups

½ cup: 2 vegetable exchanges

Protein	2 gm
Fat	0 gm
Carbohydrate	9 gm
Sodium	267 mg
Potassium	191 mg
Calories	44

¼ cup: 1 vegetable exchange

Protein	0.5 gm
Fat	0 gm
Carbohydrate	4.5 gm
Sodium	133 mg
Potassium	145 mg
Calories	20

Broccoli a la Parmesana

1 head fresh broccoli
dash of garlic powder
dash of oregano
½ tsp salt
⅛ tsp pepper
1 tbsp corn oil
2 tbsp Parmesan cheese, grated

1. Wash broccoli. Peel the stems and trim tough ends if necessary.
2. Cut into 1 inch lengths.
3. Cook broccoli in boiling salted water until tender when pierced with a fork, about 15 minutes. Drain.
4. Arrange broccoli in serving dish.
5. Sprinkle with oil, seasonings, and Parmesan cheese.
6. Serve with lemon wedges.

Yield: 6 servings
1 serving: 1 vegetable exchange

Protein	3 gm
Fat	1 gm
Carbohydrate	7 gm
Sodium	207 mg
Potassium	292 mg
Calories	49

Vegetable

4 cups celery, diced
½ lbs mushrooms, sliced
2 tbsp margarine, melted
1 tsp onion, chopped
¼ tsp salt
¼ tsp pepper

1. Place celery and mushrooms on large foil square.

2. Sprinkle with onion, salt, and pepper.

3. Drizzle with melted margarine.

4. Close foil tightly and bake at 400 degrees for one hour.

Yield: 2 cups
½ cup: 1 vegetable exchange
       1 fat exchange

Protein	2 gm
Fat	6 gm
Carbohydrate	8 gm
Sodium	360 mg
Potassium	626 mg
Calories	94

Vegetable Medley

1 onion, large, thinly sliced
1½ cups carrots, thinly sliced
¾ cup green pepper, cut in chunks
2 cups celery, sliced
2 cups green beans, frozen
2 cups stewed tomatoes, canned, broken up
2 tsp salt
dash of pepper
3 tbsp tapioca

1. Layer vegetables, except tomatoes, in flat baking dish, glass or ceramic.

2. Sprinkle tapioca and seasonings over all.

3. Spoon tomatoes and liquid over all.

4. Cover tightly with foil.

5. Bake at 350 degrees for 1 hour and 10 minutes.

Yield: 8 servings
1 serving: 2 vegetable exchanges

Protein	2 gm
Fat	0 gm
Carbohydrate	12 gm
Sodium	657 mg
Potassium	402 mg
Calories	56

Fried Rice

¼ cup chicken fat, roast pork fat, or oil
2 scallions, chopped
4 oz raw shrimp, shelled, deveined, diced
½ tsp salt
2 eggs, slightly beaten
4 oz cooked pork, diced
4 oz cooked chicken, diced
4 cups cooked rice, cold
¼ cup soy sauce
¼ tsp black pepper
⅛ tsp ground ginger
1 cup lettuce, shredded

1. Set ingredients by the stove.

2. Set wok or skillet over high heat for 30 seconds.

3. Swirl in half of the fat.

4. Add scallions, and brown lightly.

5. Add shrimp, stir-fry for 3 minutes.

6. Add salt.

7. Add eggs, scramble until not quite cooked.

8. Remove to a warm plate.

9. Swirl remaining fat into the wok.

10. Add pork and chicken, then stir-fry for 2 minutes.

11. Add rice, soy sauce, pepper, and ginger.

12. Stir and toss until heated.

13. Add scrambled eggs.

14. Stir and toss one-half minute.

15. Add lettuce.

16. Stir and toss until mixed.

17. Serve at once, before lettuce softens.

(continued)

Fried Rice (continued)

Yield: 6 servings

1 serving:	2 meat, low-fat exchanges	Protein	22 gm
	2 bread-starch exchanges	Fat	20 gm
		Carbohydrate	36 gm
		Sodium	1624 mg
	1 vegetable exchange	Potassium	302 mg
	3 fat exchanges	Calories	412

—ENTREES—
AMERICAN and
ETHNIC

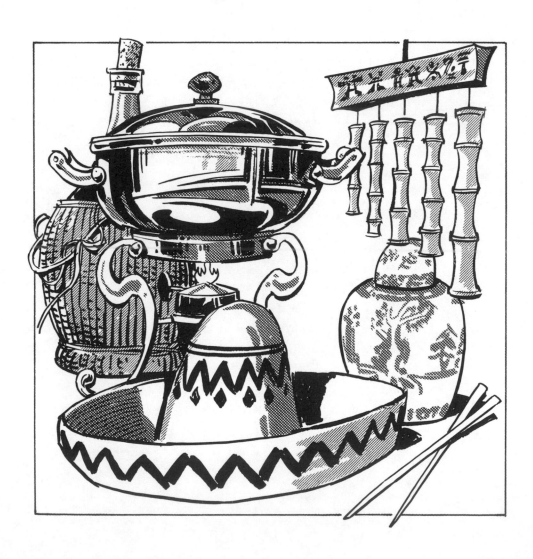

Lemon Barbecued Chicken

2 lb frying chicken
¼ cup lemon juice
¼ cup melted butter or margarine
1 small onion, grated
1 small garlic clove, minced
½ tsp salt
½ tsp celery salt
½ tsp black pepper
½ tsp rosemary
¼ tsp thyme

1. Cut chicken into 4 serving portions.

2. Marinate in barbecue mixture for several hours. (Mix remaining ingredients to make mixture.)

3. Broil, turning and brushing often with marinade until done.

Yield: 4 servings

1 serving: 4 meat, low fat exchanges	Protein	3 gm
	Fat	24 gm
2 fat exchanges	Carbohydrate	6 gm
1 vegetable exchange	Sodium	664 mg
	Potassium	365 mg
	Calories	372

Chicken Breast with Mushrooms

4 chicken breasts, halved
2 tbsp oil
1 cup mushrooms
1 can condensed cream of chicken soup
1 clove garlic, minced
1 pinch rosemary, crushed
¼ cup cream, light

1. Brown chicken breast in oil.

2. Remove from skillet.

3. Brown mushrooms.

4. Stir in soup, garlic, and seasonings.

5. Put chicken back in skillet. Pour soup over chicken and mushrooms.

6. Cover and cook over low heat for about 1 hour. Stir now and then.

Yield: 4 servings

1 serving:	4 meat, low-fat exchanges	Protein	30 gm
	½ bread-starch exchange	Fat	27 gm
		Carbohydrate	7 gm
		Sodium	600 mg
	3 fat exchanges	Potassium	145 mg
		Calories	391

Kabob of Chicken Livers

1 lb chicken livers
½ lb mushroom caps, fresh
4 tsp butter or margarine
¼ tsp salt
¼ tsp pepper
⅛ tsp onion salt

1. Alternate chicken livers and mushroom caps on skewer.

2. Brush lightly with butter or margarine. Add seasonings.

3. Broil 3 inches from flame for 10 minutes, turning often.

Yield: 4 servings

1 serving: 3 meat, low fat exchanges		
1 vegetable exchange	Protein	23 gm
	Fat	8 gm
	Carbohydrate	4 gm
	Sodium	303 mg
	Potassium	341 mg
	Calories	180

Curry Chicken

2–3 lb chicken, boiled and deboned
1 package frozen or fresh broccoli, 10 oz
1 plain, unflavored yogurt, 8 oz
1 can cream of chicken soup
1 tbsp lemon juice
1 tsp curry
4 oz cheddar cheese, grated

1. Mix yogurt, soup, lemon juice, and curry.

2. Layer the bottom of pan with broccoli, then layer chicken.

3. Pour sauce over chicken.

4. Sprinkle cheese on top.

5. Bake at 350 degrees until cheese melts (about 30 minutes).

Yield: 6 servings

1 serving:		
1 vegetable exchange	Protein	37 gm
5 meat, low-fat	Fat	20 gm
exchanges	Carbohydrate	6 gm
	Sodium	679 mg
	Potassium	201 mg
	Calories	352

Chicken a la King

8 mushrooms, sliced
½ cup clear chicken broth
2 cups skim milk
¼ cup flour
½ tsp salt
dash of pepper
1 tbsp pimento, chopped
2 cups cooked chicken, diced
4 slices toast

1. Cook fresh mushrooms in broth. Drain and measure broth, add water to make ½ cup.

2. Heat 1½ cups skim milk and ½ cup broth in the top of a double boiler.

3. Blend flour and the remaining ½ cup skim milk until no lumps remain.

4. Add to heated milk and broth, stirring constantly, until thickened (over boiling water).

5. Add chicken, mushroom, pimento, and seasoning.

6. Reheat.

Serve on toast points—1 slice cut into 4 points.

Yield: 4 servings

1 serving:	3 meat, low fat exchanges	Protein	28 gm
	1 bread-starch exchange (including toast)	Fat	10 gm
		Carbohydrate	22 gm
		Sodium	830 mg
		Potassium	379 mg
	1 vegetable exchange	Calories	290

Chicken Timbales

1¾ cups chicken, cooked and cubed
5¼ tsp margarine
⅜ cup bread crumbs
1¼ cups skim milk
5 eggs
1 tsp salt
½ tsp onion juice
½ tsp pepper

1. Mix all ingredients and add to chicken.

2. Lightly oil timbale molds and fill ¾ full or use a small loaf pan.

3. Set oven at 325 degrees. Place in pan of hot water (like a custard), and bake until firm.

4. Unmold.

Yield: 5 servings
1 serving: 4 meat, low-fat
            exchanges
        1 vegetable exchange

Serve with cream sauce and garnish with chopped parsley. See cream sauce recipe.

Protein	30 gm
Fat	14 gm
Carbohydrate	6 gm
Sodium	637 mg
Potassium	333 mg
Calories	270

Creamed Turkey

¼ **cup shortening**
1 cup flour
3 cups reconstituted non-fat dry milk
2 cups cooked or canned turkey, cubed
frozen peas, 10 oz bag
¼ **tsp salt**
¼ **tsp pepper**

1. Melt shortening, stir in flour.

2. Add milk and cook over low heat until mixture thickens.

3. Stir in turkey, vegetable, salt, and pepper. Heat thoroughly.

4. Serve over biscuit, rice, or corn bread.

Yield: 6 servings

1 serving:			
3 meat low-fat exchanges	Protein	25 gm
1 bread-starch exchange	Fat	15 gm
	Carbohydrate	23 gm
1 fat exchange	Sodium	365 mg
1 vegetable exchange	Potassium	441 mg
	Calories	327

NOTE: Add a bread-starch exchange for biscuit, rice, or corn bread.

Turkey Tetrazzini

1 box thin spaghetti (14 oz)
½ cup butter
½ cup flour
1 cup milk, 2% fat
1 can chicken broth (10¾ oz)
1 tsp salt
½ tsp pepper
¼ tsp nutmeg
¼ cup dry sherry
¾ cup light whipping cream
3 cups cooked turkey
½ lb mushrooms, sliced
3 tbsp butter
½ cup Parmesan cheese
½ cup sliced almonds

1. Cook spaghetti according to directions. Do not add salt. Drain.

2. Melt butter in large sauce pan, blend in flour, stir in milk and chicken broth.

3. Cook stirring constantly until sauce is smooth and thickened.

4. Stir in salt, pepper, nutmeg, sherry, whipping cream, and turkey.

5. Saute mushrooms in butter. Toss into drained spaghetti.

6. Spoon ½ of spaghetti into bottom of buttered 3 quart casserole.

7. Pour half of sauce over spaghetti, repeat layers.

8. Sprinkle with Parmesan cheese and almonds.

9. Bake at 350 degrees for 60–70 minutes. Let stand about 10 minutes before serving.

Yield: 3 quarts

1 cup:		
2 bread-starch exchanges	Protein	20 gm
1 meat, low fat exchange	Fat	20 gm
3 fat exchanges	Carbohydrate	32 gm
	Sodium	568 mg
	Potassium	391 mg
	Calories	388

Turkey and Ham Mornay

½ lb sliced cold breast of turkey
1½ packages broccoli spears, frozen or fresh, cooked (10 oz package) with no added salt
½ lb sliced cold roast or boiled ham, lean
2 cans cream of celery soup
⅔ soup can of water
¼ cup cracker or dry bread crumbs

1. In casserole, layer turkey, broccoli, and ham.

2. Thin soup with water and pour over layers.

3. Sprinkle crumbs carefully over top.

4. Heat in a 350 degree oven until thoroughly warmed.

Yield: 8 servings

1 serving:	2 meat, low fat exchanges	Protein	17 gm
	½ bread-starch exchange	Fat	11 gm
		Carbohydrate	10 gm
		Sodium	678 mg
	1 fat exchange	Potassium	376 mg
	1 vegetable exchange	Calories	207

Baked Fish Fillets

1 lb fish fillets, frozen or fresh
¼ cup milk, 2% fat
½ tsp salt
4 tbsp fine dry bread crumbs
4 tsp butter, bacon grease, or other fat

1. Cut fillets into 4 portions and soak 3 minutes in milk to which salt has been added.

2. Drain and roll in bread crumbs.

3. Place fish in greased baking dish and dot with fat.

4. Bake in hot oven at 450–500 degrees allowing 8 minutes if fish is fresh and 15 minutes if fish is frozen.

Yield: 4 servings

1 serving:	3 meat, low-fat exchanges	Protein	22 gm
	1 fat exchange	Fat	13 gm
	1 vegetable exchange	Carbohydrate	5 gm
		Sodium	694 mg
		Potassium	530 mg
		Calories	225

Fish Loaf

2 cups flaked fish (e.g., tuna or salmon) well drained, water
   packed
1½ cups bread crumbs
½ tsp baking powder
⅔ cup celery, chopped
⅓ cup onion, chopped
1 tbsp lemon juice
1 cup skim milk
1 tbsp pimento, minced
1 tbsp green pepper, chopped
¼ tsp salt
¼ tsp pepper

1. Mix ingredients.

2. Form loaf in an oiled loaf pan.

3. Bake in moderate oven (350 degrees) until brown and firm.

4. Serve with desired cream sauce.

Yield: 5 servings

1 serving: 3½ meat, low-fat exchanges	Protein	30 gm
1 bread-starch exchange	Fat	10 gm
1 vegetable exchange	Carbohydrate	21 gm
	Sodium	1261 mg
	Potassium	487 mg
	Calories	294

Bouillabaisse (Fish Soup)

1 medium onion, diced
12 cherry tomatoes, quartered
1 stalk celery, diced
1 bay leaf
2 tbsp tomato ketchup
¼ tsp garlic
⅛ tsp ground thyme
⅛ tsp basil
¼ tsp pepper
2 cups hot water
½ lb fresh cod fish
6 oz deveined shrimp
juice of 1 lemon
2 oz olive oil

1. Simmer first 9 ingredients for 10 minutes in 2 ounces of olive oil at medium heat.

2. Add water.

3. Broil cod about 7 minutes. Separate fish into small pieces.

4. Add shrimp and lemon juice to soup.

5. Add cod and simmer.

Yield: 6 servings

1 serving:	2 meat, low fat exchanges	Protein	16 gm
	1 bread-starch exchange	Fat	12 gm
		Carbohydrate	18 gm
		Sodium	133 mg
	1 fat exchange	Potassium	467 mg
		Calories	163

Scallops a la Huntington

1¼ lb scallops
lemon juice of 1 lemon
1 tsp oil
1 tsp parsley, finely chopped
1 tsp salt
½ tsp pepper
4 tbsp soft bread crumbs
2 tbsp Parmesan cheese, grated
1 tsp chives, finely cut

1. Clean scallops.

2. Add lemon juice, oil, parsley, salt, and pepper.

3. Cover, let stand 30 minutes.

4. Drain.

5. Mix other ingredients.

6. Dip scallops in bread crumb mixture.

7. Broil and drain.

Yield: 6 servings
1 serving: 2 meat, low fat
            exchanges

Protein	18 gm
Fat	4 gm
Carbohydrate	3 gm
Sodium	622 mg
Potassium	375 mg
Calories	120

Piquant Scallops

1 lb scallops
3 tbsp fine dry bread crumbs
8 tsp melted butter or margarine
1 tsp worcestershire sauce
2 tsp lemon juice

1. Roll scallops in the bread crumbs.

2. Arrange in 4 scallop shells or in a shallow greased baking dish.

3. Pour mixture of melted fat, worcestershire sauce and lemon juice over scallops.

4. Bake in hot oven (450 degrees to 500 degrees) for 10 minutes.

Yield: 4 servings

1 serving: 2½ meat, low-fat exchanges ½ vegetable exchange		
Protein	19 gm
Fat	9 gm
Carbohydrate	3 gm
Sodium	461 mg
Potassium	420 mg
Calories	189

Shrimp Jambolaya

12 large shrimp, cooked
1½ cups dietetic tomato sauce
½ cup green pepper and onion, chopped
1 cup canned mushrooms, sliced
1 pinch curry powder
1 cup cooked rice, no salt added

1. Simmer tomato sauce with green pepper, onion, and curry powder.

2. Add mushrooms and shrimp.

3. Serve over cooked rice.

Yield: 2 servings

1 serving:	2 meat, low-fat exchanges	Protein	22 gm
	2 bread-starch exchanges	Fat	6 gm
		Carbohydrate	43 gm
	2 vegetable exchanges	Sodium	691 mg
		Potassium	1109 mg
	OR	Calories	314
	2 meat, low-fat exchanges		
	3 bread-starch exchanges		

Lobster Boats

½ cup cooked, cold lobster, diced
½ cup cooked elbow macaroni, chilled (do not add salt to cook)
2 tbsp finely chopped onion
1 cucumber, diced
½ tsp chopped chives
⅛ tsp salt
½ tsp pepper
1 tsp mayonnaise

1. Flatten lobster tail shell as much as possible.

2. Moisten ingredients listed above with 1 tsp mayonnaise thinned with skim milk.

3. Pile salad in lobster shells.

Yield: 1 serving	Protein	17 gm
1 serving: 2 meat, low-fat	Fat	5 gm
exchanges	Carbohydrate	30 gm
2 bread-starch	Sodium	466 mg
exchanges	Potassium	674 mg
	Calories	233

Pickle Boats

1 lb ground round steak
1 tsp worcestershire sauce
½ tsp celery seed
1 egg
1 tbsp horseradish
1 medium onion, chopped
1 tsp salt
½ tsp pepper
1 dill pickle

1. Mix all ingredients but pickle together.

2. Cut pickle in quarters lengthwise, and shape hamburger mix around it in an oblong shape so as to fit a hotdog bun (small).

3. Broil about 6 minutes on each side.

4. Serve in a small hotdog bun.

Yield: 4 servings

1 serving with bun:	3 meat, medium-fat exchanges		
		Protein	25 gm
		Fat	16 gm
		Carbohydrate	18 gm
	1 bread-starch exchange	Sodium	1326 mg
		Potassium	477 mg
		Calories	316

Barbecued Hamburgers

1 lb lean ground beef
¾ cup onion, chopped
½ tsp salt
½ tsp pepper
1 can chicken gumbo soup, 10½ oz
¼ cup water
2 tbsp catsup
2 tbsp prepared mustard

1. Brown meat and onion in teflon pan. Pour off fat.

2. Add rest of the ingredients.

3. Simmer about 30 minutes.

4. Serve on 1 small hamburger bun.

Yield: 6 servings

1 serving: 2 meat, medium fat exchanges
    1 vegetable exchange

OR

    2 meat, medium fat exchanges
    1 fruit exchange

1 hamburger bun: 2 bread-starch exchanges

Protein	15 gm
Fat	11 gm
Carbohydrate	5 gm
Sodium	706 mg
Potassium	246 mg
Calories	179

Hamburger Skillet

1 lb hamburger, lean
¾ cup uncooked rice
2 tbsp oil
¼ cup onion, diced
¼ cup celery, diced
1 can tomatoes (2 lb can)
2 tsp salt
⅛ tsp pepper
1 tsp worcestershire sauce

1. Brown rice slowly in hot fat in heavy skillet, stirring frequently.

2. Add onions, celery, and hamburger; brown well. Pour off excess fat.

3. Add tomatoes and other ingredients.

4. Cover and simmer until rice is tender—about 45 minutes.

Yield: 8 servings

1 serving:	1 meat, low-fat exchange	Protein	11 gm
	1 bread-starch exchange	Fat	8 gm
		Carbohydrate	17 gm
		Sodium	687 mg
	1 fat exchange	Potassium	274 mg
		Calories	184

Shepherd's Pie

2 cups ground cooked beef
½ tsp salt
½ tsp pepper
4 tsp grated onion
1½ cups mashed potato
1 can broth or consomme

1. Add seasonings and onion to ground beef. Mix well.

2. Add consomme or broth to moisten well.

3. Thicken slightly with 1¼ tbsp flour.

4. Place in casserole dish and spread with mashed potato.

5. Bake at 350 degrees until heated through and potatoes are slightly browned.

Yield: 4 servings
1 serving: 2 meat, medium fat
        exchanges
    1 bread-starch
      exchange

Protein	20 gm
Fat	11 gm
Carbohydrate	11 gm
Sodium	1040 mg
Potassium	409 mg
Calories	223

Texas Hash

½ medium onion, sliced
1 small green pepper, minced
½ lb ground beef, lean
1 cup cooked tomatoes
⅓ cup uncooked rice
½ tsp chili powder
1 tsp salt
dash of pepper

1. Brown ground beef. Drain.

2. When almost done, add green pepper and onion. Saute.

3. Stir in remaining ingredients.

4. Pour into baking dish, cover and bake one hour.

Yield: 2 servings

1 serving:	3 meat, low fat exchanges		
		Protein	28 gm
		Fat	8 gm
	2 bread-starch exchanges	Carbohydrate	38 gm
		Sodium	1146 mg
	1 vegetable exchange	Potassium	826 mg
		Calories	336

Soy Sauce Hot Dish

1 lb lean hamburger
1 cup onion, chopped
1 cup celery, chopped
1 can mushroom soup
3 tbsp soy sauce
2 cups cooked rice

1. Brown meat in teflon pan with onions.

2. When almost done, add celery. Do not overcook; celery should be crunchy.

3. Drain off excess fat.

4. Add remaining ingredients.

5. Bake in casserole at 375 degrees for 45 minutes.

Yield: 6 servings

1 serving:	2 meat, low fat exchanges	Protein	15 gm
	1 bread-starch exchange	Fat	27 gm
		Carbohydrate	24 gm
		Sodium	1380 mg
	1 vegetable exchange	Potassium	401 mg
	4 fat exchanges	Calories	399

Five Soup Hot Dish

2 lb hamburger, lean
2 medium onions
1 can cream of celery soup
1 can cream of mushroom soup
1 can cream of chicken soup
1 can beef barley soup
1 can chicken with rice soup
1 can mushroom stems and pieces, 4 oz
8 oz chow mein noodles

1. Brown hamburger and onion together.

2. Drain off fat.

3. Add soups and mix well.

4. Fold in ⅔ of chow mein noodles.

5. Place in a large casserole or 9 x 13 inch pan.

6. Top with remaining noodles. Bake at 350 degrees for 45 minutes.

Yield: 10 servings

1 serving:	3 meat, medium fat exchanges	Protein	23 gm
	1½ bread-starch exchanges	Fat	23 gm
		Carbohydrate	25 gm
		Sodium	1211 mg
	2 fat exchanges	Potassium	356 mg
		Calories	399

Gourmet Hash

1½ cups ground cooked beef (10–11 oz raw)
1 cup ground or finely diced cooked potato
½ cup ground onion
¼ cup chopped parsley or chives
2 tbsp ground green pepper
1 tsp salt
2 tsp worcestershire sauce
⅔ cup skim milk
1 tbsp margarine

1. Mix together ingredients and turn into a greased, one quart casserole.

2. Bake at 350 degrees about 20 minutes.

Yield: 4 servings

1 serving: 2 meat, low-fat		
exchanges	Protein	14 gm
1 vegetable exchange	Fat	7 gm
	Carbohydrate	6 gm
	Sodium	831 mg
	Potassium	263 mg
	Calories	143

Six Layer Dinner

2 cups potatoes, raw, sliced
2 cups celery, chopped
1 lb lean ground beef
1 cup raw onions, sliced
1 cup green peppers, finely cut
2 cups tomatoes, canned
2 tsp salt
¼ tsp pepper
a few green pepper slices for garnish

1. Lightly oil baking dish.

2. Place ingredients in the order given in layers in an 8 x 12 inch baking dish, sprinkling salt and pepper over layers.

3. Garnish top and bake for 2 hours at 350 degrees.

Yield: 6 servings

1 serving: 2 meat, medium fat exchanges		
1 bread-starch exchange	Protein	16 gm
	Fat	11 gm
	Carbohydrate	15 gm
	Sodium	904 mg
	Potassium	745 mg
	Calories	223

Hamburger Stuffed Tomatoes

4 medium tomatoes
¾ lb lean minced beef
1 tbsp grated onion
1 tbsp chopped parsley
1 tsp worcestershire sauce
¼ cup bread crumbs
¼ cup grated cheese
¼ tsp salt
¼ tsp pepper

1. Remove stem ends of tomatoes; scoop out some of the pulp and drain tomatoes.

2. Combine beef, tomato pulp, and seasonings and stuff tomato shells with the mixture, dividing it evenly.

3. Sprinkle with mixture of bread crumbs and grated cheese.

4. Place in baking dish and bake in moderate oven (375 degrees) for 30 minutes.

Yield: 4 servings

1 serving: 2 meat, medium fat exchanges	Protein	19 gm
2 vegetable exchanges	Fat	13 gm
½ fat exchange	Carbohydrate	10 gm
	Sodium	421 mg
OR	Potassium	553 mg
	Calories	233
2 meat, medium fat exchanges		
1 fruit exchange		
½ fat exchange		

Stuffed Green Peppers

¾ lb ground beef, lean
1⅓ cup tomatoes, canned, drained
⅓ cup liquid from the tomatoes
¾ tsp salt
⅓ tsp pepper
4 green peppers, medium size
⅓ cup onion, chopped finely

1. Cook meat and onion. Drain off fat.

2. Add tomatoes, salt and pepper, and liquid. Simmer for 30 minutes in covered skillet.

3. Cut green peppers in half, remove the seeds and cook in boiling water for 3 minutes. Drain off water.

4. Fill pepper halves with mixture.

5. Arrange in greased baking dish. Add ¼ cup hot water in bottom of baking dish.

6. Bake at 350 degrees for 30 minutes.

Two pepper halves per serving.

Yield: 4 servings

1 serving: 2 meat, medium fat exchanges 2 vegetable exchanges		
Protein	17 gm
Fat	12 gm
Carbohydrate	12 gm
Sodium	562 mg
Potassium	711 mg
Calories	224

Porcupine Meatballs

1 lb hamburger
1 cup cooked rice
¼ tsp monosodium glutamate (MSG)
1-6 ounce can tomato sauce
1 cup tomato juice
½ tsp worcestershire sauce

1. Mix hamburger, rice, worcestershire sauce, and monosodium glutamate lightly.

2. Form into small balls.

3. Pour tomato sauce mixed with tomato juice over meatballs.

4. Cover. Cook in a 350 degree oven for one hour.

Yield: 4 servings

1 serving:	3 meat, medium fat exchanges	Protein	22 gm
	½ bread-starch exchange	Fat	16 gm
		Carbohydrate	18 gm
		Sodium	719 mg
	1 vegetable exchange	Potassium	556 mg
	OR	Calories	304
	3 meat, medium fat exchanges		
	1 bread-starch exchange		

Tangy Marinated Beef

2 lb well trimmed boneless round steak
¾ cup vinegar
2 large onions, chopped
3 large carrots, diced
½ tsp salt
8 peppercorns
⅛ tsp ground clove
2 bay leaves
1 tbsp cornstarch

1. Two days before serving:

   Place well trimmed meat in large bowl or pan. In saucepan combine ¾ cup water with rest of ingredients except cornstarch. Heat to boiling, then pour over the meat. Cover and refrigerate two days. Turn meat occasionally.

2. About 3 hours before serving:

   Remove meat from marinade and drain on paper towels. Pat dry. Strain and reserve marinade, discarding whole spices.

3. Brown meat on all sides in hot teflon skillet over medium heat.

4. Add marinade, cover and simmer 1 hour or until meat is tender.

5. To thicken gravy, mix cornstarch with 2 tbsp of water to form a paste. Stir into gravy and continue cooking until slightly thickened.

Yield: 8 servings

1 serving: 3 meat, medium-fat exchanges 1 vegetable exchange		
Cholesterol	7 gm
Protein	22 gm
Fat	15 gm
Carbohydrate	7 gm
Sodium	211 mg
Potassium	474 mg
Calories	251

Quickie Sauerbraten

1 lb or 2 cube steaks
½ tsp salt
⅛ tsp pepper
1 package brown gravy mix (1 oz)
1¼ cups water
½ tsp kitchen bouquet sauce
2 tbsp vinegar
1 tbsp instant minced onion
¼ tsp liquid artificial sweetener

1. Cut steaks in half.

2. Sprinkle steaks with salt and pepper.

3. Brown well over low heat.

4. Drain. Push steaks to one side.

5. Stir in mixture of gravy, water, bouquet sauce, vinegar, and onion.

6. Cover and simmer 10–15 minutes or until meat is tender.

7. Stir in liquid artificial sweetener. Serve immediately.

Yield: 4 servings
1 serving: 3 meat, medium fat exchanges, ½ fruit exchange

Protein	21 gm
Fat	15 gm
Carbohydrate	4 gm
Sodium	847 mg
Potassium	310 mg
Calories	235

Oven Beef Stew

2 lb lean chuck roast cut up, or lean stew meat
8 small raw potatoes
4 raw carrots
2 raw onions
1 can cream of mushroom soup
1 can cream of celery soup
1 package dry onion soup mix
¾ can water

1. Do not brown meat.

2. Mix all ingredients well.

3. Cover and bake 4 hours at 300 degrees.

Yield: 8 servings

1 serving:	3 meat, medium fat exchanges	Protein	23 gm
	1 bread-starch exchange	Fat	20 gm
		Carbohydrate	24 gm
		Sodium	1031 mg
	1 vegetable exchange	Potassium	776 mg
	1 fat exchange	Calories	368

Beef Stew

2 tbsp oil
3 cups mixed vegetables (carrots, peas, onions, chopped celery)
12 oz cubed beef, lean
5 cups water
½ tsp salt
pepper to taste

1. Brown beef cubes in oil.

2. Add water, salt, and pepper for seasoning.

3. Simmer slowly until meat is tender.

4. Add vegetables.

5. Cook for 30 minutes or until vegetables are done.

Yield: 6 servings

1 serving:	1½ meat, medium fat exchanges	Protein	11 gm
	1 vegetable exchange	Fat	12 gm
	1 fat exchange	Carbohydrate	7 gm
		Sodium	222 mg
		Potassium	297 mg
		Calories	180

New England Boiled Dinner

2 lb lean corned beef
4 small whole carrots
1 cup turnip, diced
4 potatoes, peeled
4 cabbage wedges
4 small onions
½ tsp pepper

1. Cover corned beef with cold water and bring to a boil.

2. Simmer in tightly covered pan for one hour.

3. Add all vegetables except cabbage and simmer ½ hour longer.

4. Add cabbage and cook uncovered for 15 minutes.

Yield: 8 servings

1 serving:	3 meat, medium fat exchanges	Protein	21 gm
	1 bread-starch exchange	Fat	16 gm
		Carbohydrate	14 gm
		Sodium	1633 mg
		Potassium	553 mg
		Calories	284

Baked Ham Patties

1 egg
2 cups ground cooked ham
1 tsp chopped onion
4 tbsp unsweetened pineapple juice
4 unsweetened, canned pineapple rings

1. Add beaten egg to ground ham.

2. Add chopped onion.

3. Season.

4. Form into 4 patties of equal size.

5. Halve pineapple slices.

6. Place 4 halves on baking dish, top with each ham patty.

7. Place remaining pineapple slices on top of ham patties.

8. Pour the pineapple juice over patties.

9. Bake in oven at 350 degrees for 15 minutes.

Yield: 4 servings
1 serving: 2 meat, high fat
          exchanges
          ½ fruit exchange

Protein	14 gm
Fat	18 gm
Carbohydrate	7 gm
Sodium	47 mg
Potassium	255 mg
Calories	246

Spanish Pork Chop

1 large onion, cut into ½ inch slices
4 large pork chops (well trimmed of fat)
1½ cups canned tomatoes
1 small green pepper, chopped
2 tsp chili powder
¼ tsp salt
¼ tsp pepper

1. Season pork chops with salt and pepper. Brown. (Sprinkle heavy frying pan with salt to prevent chops from sticking).

2. Top the chops with onion, tomatoes, green pepper, and chili powder.

3. Cover and cook slowly about 1 hour or until chops are fork tender.

Yield: 4 servings
1 serving: 3 meat, high fat
        exchanges
        1 vegetable exchange

Protein	13 gm
Fat	16 gm
Carbohydrate	8 gm
Sodium	296 mg
Potassium	524 mg
Calories	228

Stuffed Frankfurters

1 frankfurter
½ ounce cheese
1 strip of bacon (optional)

1. Cut a pocket in the frankfurter lengthwise.

2. Insert cheese, wrap with bacon.

3. Secure with toothpicks, broil until bacon is done.

Yield: 1 serving
1 serving: 1½ meat, high fat
        exchanges
        2 fat exchanges

Protein	10 gm
Fat	24 gm
Carbohydrate	1 gm
Sodium	611 mg
Potassium	119 mg
Calories	260

Lamb on Skewers

3 oz or three 1½ inch cubes cooked lamb, cut from
  shoulder or leg
2 small tomatoes (firm)
2 mushrooms, large
2 slices dill pickle
2 small onions

1. Thread pieces of lamb on skewer, alternating with mushroom,
   tomato, pickle, and onion.

2. Broil until well browned, withdrawing the skewer when ready to
   serve.

(Meat may be marinated beforehand in diluted vinegar and
rosemary.)

Yield: 1 serving

1 serving: 3 meat, medium fat exchanges 1 bread-starch exchange		
Protein	24 gm
Fat	15 gm
Carbohydrate	15 gm
Sodium	1025 mg
Potassium	970 mg
Calories	291

Cheese Souffle

¼ **cup flour**
1 tsp salt
1⅓ cups milk, 2% fat
½ tsp baking powder
6 oz sharp cheese
4 egg whites
4 egg yolks

1. Combine flour, salt, and milk in a saucepan. Cook and stir over medium heat until mixture comes to a boil.

2. Remove from heat.

3. Add cheese, stirring until melted. Cool slightly while beating eggs.

4. Beat egg whites until stiff.

5. Beat egg yolks until thick and lemon colored.

6. Add flour mixture to egg yolks. Mix well.

7. Fold in egg whites.

8. Pour into 1½ quart casserole.

9. Set in pan of hot water.

10. Bake at 375 degrees for 40 minutes or until souffle is firm. Serve at once.

Yield: 5 servings
1 serving: 2 meat, medium-fat exchanges
½ bread-starch exchange
1 fat exchange

Protein	17 gm
Fat	17 gm
Carbohydrate	8 gm
Sodium	775 mg
Potassium	174 mg
Calories	253

Cheese Fondue

1 egg, beaten
1 cup milk, 2% fat
3 slices bread, cubed
5 oz American cheese, shredded
4 tsp butter
¼ tsp salt
½ tsp pepper

1. Melt butter in skillet.

2. Add bread cubes and stir until lightly browned.

3. Place bread cubes in greased pan in alternate layers with shredded cheese.

4. Mix beaten egg, milk, salt, and pepper and pour over bread and cheese.

5. Set baking dish in pan of water (1 inch deep).

6. Bake at 350 degrees for 40 minutes. Serve hot.

Yield: 4 servings
1 serving: 2 meat, high fat
          exchanges
       1 bread-starch
          exchange

Protein	13 gm
Fat	16 gm
Carbohydrate	14 gm
Sodium	434 mg
Potassium	121 mg
Calories	252

Macaroni and Cheese

2 cups cooked macaroni
½ lb diced cheese
½ cup milk, 2% fat
¼ tsp salt
½ tsp pepper
dash of dry mustard

1. Cook cheese and milk together in double boiler until smooth.

2. Add seasonings.

3. Add macaroni and mix well. Pour into baking dish.

4. Bake in moderate (350 degrees) oven about 20 minutes or until done.

5. Serve ¾ cup of baked macaroni and cheese per serving.

Yield: 4 servings

1 serving: 2 meat, high fat exchanges
1 bread-starch exchange
½ fat exchange

Protein	17 gm
Fat	18 gm
Carbohydrate	11 gm
Sodium	793 mg
Potassium	140 mg
Calories	274

Egg and Cheese Casserole

7 slices bread, cubed (remove crust)
4 eggs, slightly beaten
½ tsp dry mustard
½ lb grated sharp cheddar cheese
2 cups skim milk
¼ tsp salt
¼ tsp pepper

1. Mix all ingredients together.

2. Turn mixture into a greased 2 quart casserole (shallow type is best).

3. Bake for 35 minutes at 350 degrees.

Yield: 6 servings

1 serving:		
1 bread-starch exchange	Protein	19 gm
	Fat	18 gm
2 meat, medium fat exchanges	Carbohydrate	18 gm
	Sodium	605 mg
2 fat exchanges	Potassium	188 mg
¼ milk exchange	Calories	310

Baked Egg Casserole

1½ dozen eggs, hard cooked, sliced thin
1 lb bacon, fried crisp and crumbly
2 cups medium white sauce
½ tsp salt
1 lb cheddar cheese, grated
1 garlic clove, crushed
¼ tsp basil
¼ tsp thyme
¼ tsp marjoram
¼ cup parsley
1 cup cheese croutons

WHITE SAUCE
2 tbsp butter
2 tbsp flour
¼ tsp salt
1 cup skim milk

1. To make white sauce, melt butter, blend flour and salt. Add milk. Cook quickly, stirring until sauce thickens and bubbles. Remove from heat.

2. Add cheese and spices to white sauce. Heat slowly until cheese melts.

3. Pour part of sauce into greased oblong pan.

4. Add layer of eggs and crumbled bacon.

5. Repeat in layers steps 3 and 4 above.

6. Top with croutons.

7. Bake in 19 x 13 inch pan at 350 degrees for 25 minutes or until bubbly and crumbs have browned.

Yield: 15 servings (3 x 2½ inch square)

1 serving: 2½ meat, medium fat		
exchanges	Protein	19 gm
4 fat exchanges	Fat	35 gm
	Carbohydrate	2 gm
	Sodium	632 mg
	Potassium	182 mg
	Calories	399

Baked Lasagna

4 cups canned tomatoes
1-8 oz can tomato sauce
1 tsp salt
1½ tsp onion salt
⅛ tsp pepper
1 lb lean ground beef
½ lb lasagna noodles
1 egg
2 cups cottage cheese
½ lb grated mozarella cheese
½ cup Parmesan cheese
1½ tsp oregano

1. Combine in saucepan: tomatoes, tomato sauce, salt, oregano, onion salt, and pepper. Simmer mixture uncovered.

2. Brown ground beef until meat loses its red color. Drain fat and add to sauce. Simmer for 2½ hours.

3. Cook lasagna noodles. One-half tsp oil added to water prevents noodles from sticking. Drain.

4. Mix cottage cheese with beaten egg.

5. Grate mozarella cheese and Parmesan cheese.

6. Layer items: cover bottom of 9 x 13 inch pan with ¼ inch of meat sauce. Add ½ of the noddles on top. Add ½ cottage cheese mixture, ⅓ of the mozarella cheese, and ½ of the Parmesan·cheese.

7. Repeat layers, ending with meat sauce, topped with mozarella cheese.

8. Bake until bubbly (30–35 minutes), covered.

9. Remove from oven and let stand 15 minutes.

Yield: 8 servings

1 serving:	4 meat, low fat exchanges	Protein	33 gm
	2 bread-starch exchanges	Fat	20 gm
		Carbohydrate	31 gm
		Sodium	1010 mg
	2 fat exchanges	Potassium	628 mg
		Calories	436

(continued)

Baked Lasagna (continued)

Yield: 16 servings

1 serving:	2 meat, low fat exchanges	Protein	16 gm
	1 bread-starch exchange	Fat	10 gm
	1 fat exchange	Carbohydrate	15 gm
		Sodium	505 mg
		Potassium	314 mg
		Calories	214

Italian Spaghetti

4 tsp oil
8 tsp onion, chopped fine
½ cup tomato puree
1 cup water
2 cups tomatoes, canned
¾ lb ground beef
2 cups spaghetti, cooked
¼ tsp salt
pepper to taste

---

1. Cook meat, drain off fat. Measure fat back into pan.

2. Brown onion in fat.

3. Add the tomato paste, water, tomatoes, and seasonings.

4. Simmer all gently for one hour. If needed, add more water.

5. Serve on cooked spaghetti. One or two teaspoons of grated Parmesan cheese may be used per serving.

Yield: 4 servings

1 serving:	2 meat, medium fat exchanges	Protein	19 gm
	1 bread-starch exchange	Fat	17 gm
	1 fat exchange	Carbohydrate	23 gm
	1 vegetable exchange	Sodium	442 mg
		Potassium	611 mg
		Calories	321

Manicotti

Manicotti shells

1. Cook 12 shells according to directions on package.
2. Drain and cool.

Bechamel Sauce

3 tbsp polyunsaturated margarine
3 tbsp flour
½ tsp salt
2¼ cups fluid skim milk
¼ tsp nutmeg

---

1. Melt margarine in top of double boiler.

2. Stir in flour, salt and nutmeg.

3. Cook, stirring, over low heat until the mixture is thickened and shiny.

4. Add milk gradually, stirring to prevent lumps.

5. Place over boiling water and cook, stirring constantly, until the sauce is thickened and begins to boil.

6. Remove from heat and set aside.

Filling

¼ cup margarine
1 cup celery, finely minced
½ cup onion, finely minced
½ cup mushrooms (fresh), minced
1 pound ground veal
1 tsp salt
dash of pepper
½ cup dry bread crumbs
2 egg yolks, medium size
1 tbsp tomato paste
¼ cup white wine (dry)
1-10 ounce can mild spaghetti sauce

(continued)

Manicotti (continued)

1. Melt margarine in skillet or saute pan.

2. Add minced vegetables, veal, salt, and pepper.

3. Saute until the meat is lightly browned and the vegetables are limp.

4. Cover and cook over low heat about 20 minutes.

5. Remove from heat.

6. Add bread crumbs, egg yolks, tomato paste, and wine to the mixture.

7. Combine to distribute ingredients evenly.

To assemble manicotti shells, bechamel sauce, and filling:

1. Preheat oven to 400 degrees.

2. Spray a casserole (2 quart square) or 9 x 12 inch baking pan with non-stick shortening substitute.

3. Layer half the bechamel sauce on the bottom of the pan.

4. Top with half of the spaghetti sauce.

5. Spoon the filling carefully into the manicotti shells (or use an icing tube), being certain not to use too much pressure which would break the pasta.

6. Arrange the stuffed manicotti on the sauces. Top with the remaining bechamel and spaghetti sauces.

7. Bake uncovered for 30 minutes.

8. Remove from oven and let stand 15 minutes before serving.

Yield: 6 servings
     (2 manicotti each)

1 serving:	3 meat, medium fat exchanges	Protein	27 gm
	3 bread-starch exchanges	Fat	27 gm
		Carbohydrate	43 gm
		Sodium	1003 mg
	2 fat exchanges	Potassium	688 mg
		Calories	523

12 servings (1 manicotti each)

1 serving:	1½ meat, medium fat exchange	Protein	14 gm
	1 bread-starch exchange	Fat	14 gm
		Carbohydrate	21 gm
		Sodium	501 mg
	1 vegetable exchange	Potassium	344 mg
	1 fat exchange	Calories	266

Pizza Burgers

1½ lb ground beef
½ cup diced onion
½ cup diced green pepper
1 quart Italian spaghetti sauce
¼ tsp paprika
1 tsp worcestershire sauce
¼ tsp garlic salt
½ tsp oregano

1. Brown ground beef.

2. Add onion and green pepper.

3. Saute until vegetables are tender.

4. Add remaining ingredients.

5. Simmer for one hour.

6. Add ¼ cup meat sauce to one-half of an English muffin.

Serving size: ½ English muffin:		
1 meat, medium fat exchange	Protein	9 gm
	Fat	5 gm
	Carbohydrate	19 gm
	Sodium	329 mg
1 bread-starch exchange	Potassium	249 mg
½ fruit exchange	Calories	157

Taco Salad

1 lb hamburger, lean
2 tsp chili powder
1 lb cheddar cheese, grated
1-16 oz can kidney beans (drained)
4 tomatoes, diced
1 medium onion, grated
1 large head of lettuce, torn
1-8½ oz bag taco chips, crushed
1 cup catalina dressing

1. Brown hamburger. Drain fat.

2. Drain hamburger by putting it in a strainer and rinse under water.

3. Season with chili powder and pepper.

4. Toss all ingredients together with salad dressing.

Yield: 16 servings
1 serving
(about 1 cup):

1 bread-starch exchange	Protein	15 gm
	Fat	27 gm
2 meat, medium-fat exchanges	Carbohydrate	19 gm
	Sodium	687 mg
3 fat exchanges	Potassium	460 mg
	Calories	379

Tacos

12 tortillas
3 cups lettuce, shredded
2 large tomatoes, sliced
6 oz cheddar cheese, grated

1. Drop tortillas in hot oil, one at a time.

2. After a few seconds, turn, fold in half, and fry to desired crispness.

3. Drain well on paper towels and keep warm in a low-heat oven.

4. To serve, open each tortilla gently and insert filling.

Yield: 12 servings
1 serving (without the meat or
chicken filling): ½ meat, high fat

exchange	Protein	6 gm
1 bread-starch	Fat	4 gm
exchange	Carbohydrate	16 gm
	Sodium	233 mg
	Potassium	149 mg
	Calories	124

Refried Beans

2 tbsp bacon fat
2 cups cooked Mexican beans

1. Heat bacon fat in frying pan.

2. Add beans and a little of the liquid from the frying pan.

3. Mash well.

4. Fry the beans for a few minutes, turning to prevent burning, until they form a thick paste.

Yield: 2 cups
1 serving (½ cup): 1 bread-starch

exchange	Protein	4 gm
1 fat exchange	Fat	6 gm
	Carbohydrate	18 gm
	Sodium	3 mg
	Potassium	299 mg
	Calories	142

Taco Filling (Chicken)

2 cups cooked chicken, shredded (about 12 oz)
2 tbsp margarine
1 envelope commercial taco flavoring
2 canned green chilis, diced
2 onions, chopped
½ cup fresh tomatoes, peeled and chopped

1. Mix all ingredients and saute in margarine.

Yield: filling for 12 tacos

1 serving: 1 meat, lean exchange

Protein	7 gm
Fat	4 gm
Carbohydrate	2 gm
Sodium	16 mg
Potassium	207 mg
Calories	72

Taco with chicken filling, lettuce, tomato, and 1 tsp cheese.

1 taco: 1 bread-starch exchange
1½ meat, medium fat
exchanges

OR

1 bread-starch exchange
1½ meat, low-fat
exchange
1 fat exchange

Protein	13 gm
Fat	8 gm
Carbohydrate	18 gm
Sodium	249 mg
Potassium	356 mg
Calories	196

Taco Filling (Beef)

1 tbsp cooking oil
½ onion, minced
1 garlic clove, minced
1 lb lean ground beef
1 envelope commercial taco flavoring
½ tsp salt
pepper to taste

1. Saute onions and garlic in oil.

2. Add meat.

3. Brown.

4. Add other ingredients.

Yield: Filling for 12 tacos.

1 serving: 1 meat, low-fat exchange		
	Protein	6 gm
½ fat exchange	Fat	6 gm
	Carbohydrate	0 gm
OR	Sodium	149 mg
	Potassium	84 mg
1 meat, medium fat exchange	Calories	78

Taco with meat filling, lettuce, tomato, and 1 tbsp cheese.

1 taco: 1½ meat, medium fat exchanges		
	Protein	12 gm
	Fat	10 gm
1 bread-starch exchange	Carbohydrate	16 gm
OR	Sodium	382 mg
	Potassium	233 mg
1½ meat, low-fat exchanges	Calories	202
1 bread-starch exchange		
1 fat exchange		

Tostados

8 tortillas
oil for frying
2 cups refried beans
2 cups meat filling
2 cups shredded lettuce
2 sliced tomatoes
1 cup sliced avocado
½ cup Parmesan cheese, packed lightly
1 pint sour cream
¼ cup olives (about 8 ripe olives), sliced
pickled chili slices

1. Fry tortillas on both sides in hot oil until crisp.

2. Drain well on paper towels.

3. Spread tortillas generously with refried beans, then meat filling.

4. Add lettuce, tomato, and avocado.

5. Sprinkle with Parmesan cheese.

6. Top with sour cream.

7. Add pickled chili slices and olives.

Yield: 8 servings

1 serving:	2 meat, medium fat exchanges		Protein	13 gm
	1 vegetable exchange		Fat	28 gm
	3 fat exchanges		Carbohydrate	8 gm
			Sodium	407 mg
	OR		Potassium	150 mg
			Calories	336
	2 meat, medium fat exchanges			
	½ bread-starch exchange			
	3 fat exchanges			

Meat Filling

½ pound ground beef
½ cup onion, chopped
1 tbsp oil
4 tbsp canned green chilis, chopped
1 cup canned tomatoes, drained
½ tsp salt
⅛ tsp oregano

1. Brown meat, onion, and garlic in hot oil.

2. Add the remaining ingredients.

3. Simmer for 30 minutes, stirring frequently to prevent burning.

Yield: 3 cups
1 serving (½ cup): 1 meat,

1 meat, medium fat exchange	Protein	7 gm
	Fat	8 gm
	Carbohydrate	3 gm
½ vegetable exchange	Sodium	291 mg
	Potassium	183 mg
½ fat exchange	Calories	112

Texas Chili

1 lb ground beef, lean
2 tbsp margarine or oil
1 large onion sliced
1 green pepper, chopped
1 can kidney beans, 20 oz size
2 cups tomatoes, fresh
8 oz can seasoned tomato sauce
1½ tbsp chili powder
1½ tsp salt
a few grains of pepper
1 bay leaf
dash of paprika

1. Brown meat, onion, and green pepper in the meat fat.

2. Drain off the fat. Add beans, tomatoes, sauce, bay leaf, and seasonings.

3. Cook below boiling for ½ hour. Tastes better if made the day before and reheated.

Yield: 6 servings

1 serving:	2 meat, low fat exchanges	Protein	19 gm
	2 bread-starch exchanges	Fat	10 gm
		Carbohydrate	23 gm
		Sodium	781 mg
	2 fat exchanges	Potassium	808 mg
		Calories	258

Chili Con Carne

1½ cups raw hamburger, lean
2 tbsp chopped onion
3 cups canned tomatoes
4 drops tabasco sauce
1 tsp salt
1 cup canned red kidney beans

1. Brown hamburger, stirring to separate meat. Drain.

2. Add onion, canned tomatoes, tabasco sauce and salt.

3. Cover and simmer 1 hour, stirring occasionally.

4. Add kidney beans and reheat before serving.

Yield: 4 servings
1 serving: 3 meat, low-fat
         exchanges
     1 bread-starch
         exchange

Protein	22 gm
Fat	9 gm
Carbohydrate	17 gm
Sodium	856 mg
Potassium	830 mg
Calories	237

Beef Chow Mein

¾ lb ground beef
4 tsp fat
4 tbsp onions, chopped fine
1⅓ cup celery, thinly sliced
1⅓ cup Chinese vegetables
2 cups hot water
1 tsp salt
4 tsp cornstarch
1 cup cold water
4 tbsp soy sauce
2 cups cooked rice

1. Brown meat, drain off fat.

2. Measure fat into pan, brown onion.

3. Add celery, Chinese vegetables, hot water, salt, and soy sauce; simmer 15–20 minutes.

4. Combine cornstarch with cold water, add to mixture, cook until thickened, stirring continuously.

5. Serve ¾ cup over ½ cup rice per serving.

Yield: 4 servings

1 serving: 2 meat, medium fat exchanges	Protein	18 gm
2 bread-starch exchanges	Fat	12 gm
	Carbohydrate	39 gm
	Sodium	2333 mg
1 fruit exchange	Potassium	589 mg
	Calories	336

Chow Mein

¾ lb veal steak
¾ lb lean pork
2 tbsp oil
1 cup onion, sliced
3 cups celery, cut in diagonal strips
2 cups boiling water
1-28 oz can Chinese vegetables
2 bouillon cubes
4 oz can mushrooms
¼ cup cornstarch
½ cup water
2 tbsp soy sauce
1 tbsp dark molasses
1 tsp salt

1. Cut meat into thin strips. Brown lightly in oil.

2. Add onions, water, and seasoning including bouillon cubes. Cover tightly and simmer 20 minutes or until meat is almost tender.

3. Add celery, bean sprouts, and mushrooms. Cook 3 minutes covered tightly.

4. Make a paste of cornstarch and water. Stir into meat and vegetable mixture. Continue to stir gently until mixture is thickened (about 2 minutes).

5. Serve on Chinese noodles.

Yield: 8 servings

1 serving:			
1 bread-starch exchange	Protein	15 gm
2 meat, low-fat exchanges	Fat	16 gm
	Carbohydrate	15 gm
2 fat exchanges	Sodium	714 mg
	Potassium	676 mg
	Calories	264

½ cup Chinese noodles:
  1 bread-starch exchange
  1 fat exchange

Chop Suey

2 tbsp oil
1 medium onion, chopped
1 clove of garlic, peeled and minced
4 medium stalks celery, thin strips
1 medium sweet pepper, thin strips
1 cup bean sprouts, drained
½ lb mushrooms
1 lb beef
1 tbsp soy sauce
1 tbsp cornstarch
¼ cup water

1. Use wok or large cast iron skillet.

2. Cut celery, sweet pepper, and mushrooms into thin strips.

3. Cut beef into 2 inch thin strips.

4. Mix cornstarch with water.

5. Set wok or skillet over high heat.

6. Add oil.

7. Add each ingredient separately. Stir fry each one minute before adding the next ingredients: onion and garlic, celery, green pepper, and bean sprouts.

8. Push vegetables to sides of wok or skillet.

9. Push mushrooms to one side. Add beef and stir until warmed through.

10. Sprinkle soy sauce over ingredients.

11. Add cornstarch mixture.

12. Mix all ingredients until sauce is thick and clear. Serve at once.

Yield: 6 servings

1 serving: 2 meat, medium fat exchanges	Protein	14 gm
1 bread-starch exchange	Fat	16 gm
	Carbohydrate	13 gm
	Sodium	321 mg
1 fat exchange	Potassium	613 mg
with ½ cup rice: 1 bread-starch exchange	Calories	252

Sukiyaki

1 lb steak
¼ tsp paprika
2 tbsp butter or margarine
⅔ cup soy sauce
⅓ cup water
1 tsp monosodium glutamate (MSG)
1 tsp liquid artificial sweetener
1 cup green onions, cut into strips
2 cups sliced fresh mushrooms
1 lb can bean sprouts, drained
5 oz can bamboo shoots, drained
5 oz can water chestnuts, drained and sliced

1. Cut meat into thin slices across the grain: 1 inch wide and 2 inches long.

2. Sprinkle meat with paprika.

3. Brown in butter 2–3 minutes.

4. Pour mixture of soy sauce, water, monosodium glutamate, and liquid sweetener over meat.

5. Push meat to one side of skillet or wok. Keep ingredients separate, add green onions and fresh mushrooms.

6. Cover and cook over medium heat for 3–5 minutes.

7. Add bean sprouts, bamboo shoots and water chestnuts.

8. Cook for 4–5 minutes. *Do not overcook.*

9. Serve over rice (½ cup cooked rice per serving). (Do not add salt to rice when cooking.)

Yield: 6 servings

1 serving:	2 meat, medium-fat exchanges	Protein	18 gm
	1½ bread-starch exchanges	Fat	20 gm
		Carbohydrate	28 gm
		Sodium	2636 mg
	1 vegetable exchange	Potassium	756 mg
	2 fat exchanges	Calories	364

Egg Rolls

2 tbsp vegetable oil
2 cups shredded raw cabbage
1 large stalk celery, minced
5 oz cooked pork, chopped fine
5 oz raw shrimp, shelled, deveined, chopped
1 tbsp minced onion
1½ tsp salt
⅛ tsp grated black pepper
2½ tsp sugar
10 egg roll wrappers
1 egg, slightly beaten
3 cups oil
Chinese mustard
sweet-and-sour sauce

1. Swirl two tablespoons of oil in a hot wok or skillet.

2. Add cabbage and celery. Stir-fry for 2 minutes. Remove pan from heat.

3. Add the pork, shrimp, scallions, salt, pepper, and sugar. Mix.

4. Fill rolls.

5. Roll and seal with egg.

6. Let rolls rest 1 hour on oiled wax paper.

7. Heat wok or skillet.

8. Fry rolls in 3 cups of oil.

9. Drain and keep warm until ready to serve.

10. Serve with mustard and sweet-and-sour sauce.

Yield: 10 servings

1 serving:	1 meat, medium fat exchange	Protein	9 gm
		Fat	11 gm
	1 bread-starch exchange	Carbohydrate	17 gm
		Sodium	475 mg
	1 fat exchange	Potassium	112 mg
		Calories	203

NOTE: Mustard and sweet-and-sour sauce will add sodium and calories.

Basic Crepe

1¼ cup flour
pinch of salt
3 eggs beaten
1½ cup milk, 2% fat
2 tbsp butter, melted

1. Place all ingredients in blender or mixer and beat well.

2. Let batter stand for 1 hour for more perfect crepes.

Yield: 26 crepes

one crepe: ½ bread-starch exchange
½ fat exchange

Protein	2 gm
Fat	2 gm
Carbohydrate	6 gm
Sodium	31 mg
Potassium	35 mg
Calories	50

two crepes: 1 bread-starch exchange
1 fat exchange

Protein	4 gm
Fat	4 gm
Carbohydrate	12 gm
Sodium	62 mg
Potassium	70 mg
Calories	100

Quiche

1 egg
¾ cup all-purpose flour
1 tsp Parmesan cheese, grated
1 cup milk, 2% fat
1 cup (4 oz) Swiss cheese, shredded
½ tsp salt
⅛ tsp pepper
½ tsp oregano

1. Combine egg, flour, Parmesan cheese, ½ cup milk, and seasonings.

2. Beat until smooth.

3. Blend in remaining milk.

4. Stir in half of Swiss cheese.

5. Pour into pan.

6. Bake at 425 degrees for 30 minutes.

7. Sprinkle remaining cheese over top.

8. Bake until cheese is melted, about 2 minutes.

Yield: 4 servings

1 serving: 2 meat, medium fat
exchanges
1 bread-starch
exchange
1 fruit exchange

OR

½ cup milk, 2% fat
1 bread-starch
exchange
1 meat, medium fat
exchange
½ fat exchange

Protein	14 gm
Fat	11 gm
Carbohydrate	23 gm
Sodium	770 mg
Potassium	158 mg
Calories	247

Turkey Quiche

9 inch pie shell, unbaked
½ cup chopped onion
½ cup sliced mushrooms
1 tbsp margarine
8 oz or 2 cups aged Swiss or Gruyere cheese, grated
4 oz turkey, cooked and cubed
4 eggs, slightly beaten
2 cups milk, 2% fat
1 tsp salt
¼ tsp nutmeg
⅛ tsp cayenne or black pepper
1 tbsp flour

1. Prick and bake pie crust until lightly browned, about 5 minutes.

2. Saute mushrooms and onions in fat.

3. Sprinkle mushrooms and onions and turkey over crust.

4. Top with grated cheese.

5. Mix eggs, milk, flour, salt, nutmeg, and pepper together. Pour into pie shell.

6. Bake at 375 degrees for 45–50 minutes or until a knife comes out clean.

Yield: 8 servings

1 serving:	2 meat, medium fat exchanges	Protein	19 gm
	1 bread-starch exchange	Fat	22 gm
		Carbohydrate	13 gm
		Sodium	703 mg
	2 fat exchanges	Potassium	247 mg
		Calories	326

DESSERTS

Fruit, Pudding/Custard, Pie, Cake, Cookies, Candy

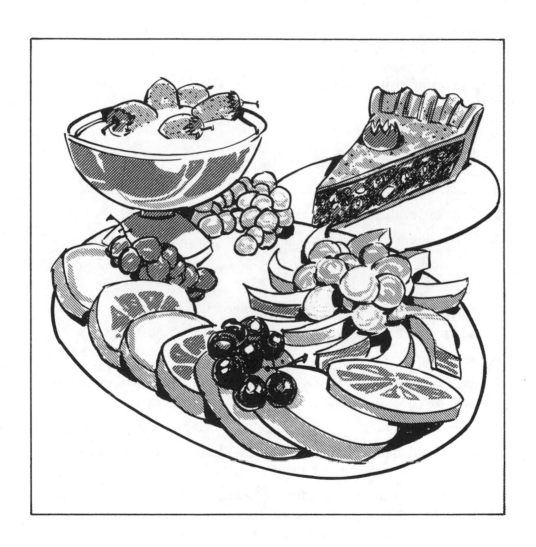

Regal Plum Pudding

4 slices bread, torn in pieces
1 cup milk, whole
6 oz beef suet, ground
1 cup packed brown sugar
2 beaten eggs
¼ cup orange juice
1 tsp vanilla
2 cups raisins
1 cup snipped pitted dates
½ cup diced, mixed candied fruits and peels
½ cup chopped walnuts
1 cup all-purpose flour
2 tsp ground cinnamon
1 tsp ground cloves
1 tsp ground mace
1 tsp baking soda
½ tsp salt
Foamy Sauce (optional)

1. Soak bread in milk; beat the bread up.

2. Stir in ground suet, brown sugar, eggs, orange juice, and vanilla.

3. In a large bowl combine raisins, dates, candied fruits and peels, and nuts.

4. Stir together the flour, cinnamon, cloves, mace, soda, and salt.

5. Add to the fruit mixture and mix well.

6. Stir in bread-suet mixture. Mix well.

7. Pour into well greased 2-quart mold (do not use a ring mold or tube pan).

8. Cover the mold with foil and tie foil on tightly with a string.

9. Place the mold on a rack in a deep kettle. Add boiling water to the kettle to a depth of 1 inch.

10. Cover and steam the pudding 3½ hours. Add more boiling water when needed.

11. Cool the pudding about 10 minutes.

12. Remove from the mold.

(continued)

Regal Plum Pudding (continued)

13. Serve the pudding with Foamy Sauce, if desired.

Yield: 16

1 serving: 3 bread-starch exchanges	Protein	8 gm
2½ fat exchanges	Fat	13 gm
	Carbohydrate	48 gm
	Sodium	157 mg
	Potassium	318 mg
	Calories	341

½ serving: 1 bread-starch exchange	Protein	4 gm
1 fruit exchange	Fat	6 gm
1 fat exchange	Carbohydrate	24 gm
	Sodium	78 mg
	Potassium	159 mg
	Calories	160

Tapioca Pudding

1 cup whole milk
1 tbsp quick-cooking tapioca
¼ tsp vanilla
liquid artificial sweetener to taste

1. Mix tapioca and milk in top of a double boiler.

2. Heat, stirring constantly until milk comes to a boil.

3. Remove from heat.

4. Add vanilla and liquid artificial sweetener.

5. Chill and serve.

Yield: 1 serving

1 serving: ½ bread-starch exchange	Protein	8 gm
1 whole milk exchange	Fat	10 gm
	Carbohydrate	19 gm
	Sodium	122 mg
	Potassium	353 mg
	Calories	198

Old Fashioned Rice Pudding

2 tbsp rice, uncooked
1 cup whole milk
1 tsp vanilla
¼ tsp cinnamon
liquid artificial sweetener to taste

1. Wash the rice.

2. Place in a large size individual casserole.

3. Pour ½ cup of milk over the rice.

4. Set the dish in a pan of water.

5. Place in a moderate oven.

6. Allow to bake until a brown crust forms.

7. With a spoon, turn the crust under and mix with rice. Do this 2 or 3 times during the baking.

8. As the milk is absorbed by the cooking rice, pour the remaining milk into the dish.

9. During the last part of the cooking, add the vanilla and cinnamon.

10. As soon as the rice is soft, remove from the oven, and chill.

Optional: 2 tbsp of raisins may be added at step 9.

Yield: 1 serving	Protein	10 gm
1 serving: 1 fruit exchange	Fat	10 gm
1 milk exchange	Carbohydrate	22 gm
Add 1 fruit exchange if raisins are	Sodium	122 mg
added.	Potassium	373 mg
	Calories	218

Rice Pudding

1 cup regular rice
2 cups water
1½ quart of whole milk
3 eggs
¾ cup sugar
1 tsp salt
¼ tsp nutmeg
⅔ cup raisins

1. Rinse rice in hot water. Boil down with 2 cups water. Do not drain.

2. Add scalded milk and cook 30 minutes.

3. Beat eggs in large bowl.

4. Mix in sugar and salt. Stir in rice and raisins slowly.

5. Pour into baking dish.

6. Place dish in pan of water before putting in oven.

7. Bake at 300 degrees for 45 minutes.

8. Stir rice once or twice while baking then top with nutmeg.

Yield: 2½ quarts

½ cup:	1 bread-starch exchange	Protein	5 gm
	½ meat, high fat exchange	Fat	4 gm
		Carbohydrate	16 gm
		Sodium	142 mg
		Potassium	126 mg
		Calories	120
1 cup:	1 bread-starch exchange	Protein	9 gm
	1½ fruit exchanges	Fat	8 gm
	1 meat, medium fat exchange	Carbohydrate	32 gm
		Sodium	284 mg
	½ fat exchange	Potassium	250 mg
		Calories	236

Indian Pudding

3 cups whole milk
½ cup molasses
⅓ cup yellow cornmeal
½ tsp ground ginger
½ tsp ground cinnamon
¼ tsp salt
1 tbsp butter

1. In saucepan, mix milk and molasses.

2. Stir in cornmeal, ginger, cinnamon, and salt.

3. Cook and stir until thick, about 10 minutes.

4. Stir in butter.

5. Turn into a 1-quart casserole.

6. Bake, uncovered, at 300 degrees for about 1 hour.

Yield: 6 servings

1 serving:			
1 bread-starch exchange	Protein	5 gm
1 fat exchange	Fat	7 gm
1 fruit exchange	Carbohydrate	26 gm
½ meat, low-fat exchange	Sodium	199 mg
	Potassium	976 mg
	Calories	187

Bread Pudding

1 cup raisins
3 cups skim milk
6 eggs
½ cup sugar
1 tsp vanilla
1 tsp nutmeg
1 tsp cinnamon
6 slices bread, broken up
1 tbsp margarine

1. Grease pan with margarine.

2. Soak raisins in water.

3. Layer bread on bottom of pan.

4. Heat milk, add raisins.

5. Beat eggs, sugar, and vanilla. Add cinnamon and nutmeg.

6. Pour egg mixture and milk over bread.

7. Bake at 350 degrees in 9x13 inch pan. Pudding is done when knife is inserted and comes out clean.

Yield: 15 servings

1 serving:	1 bread-starch exchange	Protein	7 gm
	½ fruit exchange	Fat	3 gm
	½ meat, medium fat exchange	Carbohydrate	23 gm
		Sodium	114 mg
		Potassium	184 mg
		Calories	147

Floating Island Pudding

½ cup milk*
1 egg
¼ tsp vanilla
liquid artificial sweetener to taste

1. Heat milk in top part of a double boiler.

2. Separate the egg. Beat the egg yolk well.

3. Pour the hot milk over the yolk.

4. Mix well and pour back into the double boiler.

5. In about 10 minutes the mixture will begin to thicken and will coat a spoon. Stir constantly during this time.

6. Remove from heat.

7. Add vanilla and artificial sweetener.

8. Chill.

9. Beat egg white stiff with rotary beater.

10. Chill.

11. When ready to serve the custard, place in a glass dish and top with beaten egg white.

12. Place under broiler and brown for a few seconds.

Yield: 1 serving
1 serving: ½ milk exchange
        2 fat exchanges

Protein	7 gm
Fat	11 gm
Carbohydrate	6 gm
Sodium	122 mg
Potassium	240 mg
Calories	151

*If skim milk is used, 1 serving: ½ milk exchange
                                1 fat exchange

Lemon Pudding

2⅔ tbsp cornstarch
¼ cup cold water
3 cups boiling water
¼ cup lemon juice
1 tbsp liquid artificial sweetener
1 tsp lemon rind, grated

1. Blend cornstarch and cold water.

2. Mix boiling water with mixture. Boil 3 minutes stirring constantly.

3. Add lemon juice, rind, and liquid artificial sweetener.

4. Pour each individual serving over crumbs of graham cracker in sherbet glass.

5. Sprinkle part of crumbs on top.

Yield: 6 servings
1 serving: ½ fruit exchange

Protein	0 gm
Fat	0 gm
Carbohydrate	4 gm
Sodium	0 mg
Potassium	15 mg
Calories	16

Custard Sauce

1 cup milk
1 egg yolk, beaten
1 tsp liquid artificial sweetener
dash of vanilla

1. Combine all ingredients.

2. Cook on top part of a double boiler until mixture coats a spoon.

Yield: 2 servings

1 serving: ½ milk exchange		
½ fat exchange	Protein	5 gm
	Fat	8 gm
	Carbohydrate	6 gm
	Sodium	64 mg
	Potassium	181 mg
	Calories	116

Almond Bark Cookies

2 cups peanuts
2 cups small marshmallows
2 cups Captain Crunch cereal
2 cups Rice Krispies
2 lbs almond bark candy

1. Melt almond bark and marshmallows.

2. Add rest of ingredients. Mix well.

3. Drop by teaspoonfuls onto foil.

Yield: 4 dozen (48) cookies

1 cookie: 1 bread-starch exchange		
1 fat exchange	Protein	2 gm
	Fat	5 gm
	Carbohydrate	19 gm
	Sodium	88 mg
	Potassium	67 mg
	Calories	129

Baked Custard

1 cup milk
2 eggs
a few grains of salt
¾ tsp liquid artificial sweetener
¼ tsp vanilla
dash of nutmeg

1. Scald milk.

2. Beat eggs.

3. Add salt and pour eggs slowly into the slightly coated scalded milk.

4. Add liquid artificial sweetener and vanilla.

5. Pour into custard cups.

6. Sprinkle with nutmeg.

7. Set the cups in a pan of hot water and bake for about 45 minutes at 325 degrees.

Yield: 2 servings
1 serving: 1 meat, medium-fat

exchange	Protein	10 gm
½ milk exchange	Fat	11 gm
	Carbohydrate	6 gm
	Sodium	172 mg
	Potassium	240 mg
	Calories	163

Maple Crumb Custard

2 eggs, slightly beaten
2 tsp liquid artificial sweetener
2 tsp vanilla extract
¼ tsp salt
2 cups skim milk
2 drops yellow food coloring
3 tbsp graham cracker crumbs
1 tbsp butter, melted
½ tsp maple flavoring

1. Combine in mixing bowl, eggs, liquid artificial sweetener, vanilla extract, and salt.

2. Stir in milk and food coloring.

3. Pour into 1-quart baking dish.

4. Place in pan filled 1 inch deep with hot water.

5. Bake at 350 degrees for 30 minutes.

6. Sprinkle mixture of graham cracker crumbs, butter, and maple flavoring over top.

7. Bake until knife inserted 1 inch from edge comes out clean, about 5 minutes.

8. Serve warm or chilled.

Yield: 6 servings

1 serving: ¼ skim milk exchange		
½ fat exchange	Protein	3 gm
	Fat	3 gm
OR	Carbohydrate	3 gm
	Sodium	190 mg
¼ whole milk exchange	Potassium	149 mg
	Calories	51

Pumpkin Custard

1 cup pumpkin, cooked or canned
1 egg
½ cup skim milk
⅜ tsp cinnamon
⅛ tsp ginger
⅛ tsp cloves
⅛ tsp nutmeg
1½ tsp liquid artificial sweetener

1. Beat the eggs and combine with the liquid artificial sweetener.

2. Add the milk and mix well.

3. Add the spices.

4. Pour into pan.

5. Bake in a moderate oven (350 degrees) for 50–60 minutes.

6. Test by inserting a knife near the edge. When it comes out clean, the custard is done.

Yield: 3 servings

1 serving: ½ meat, medium-fat exchange		
1 vegetable exchange	Protein	5 gm
OR	Fat	2 gm
½ cup skim milk exchange	Carbohydrate	7 gm
½ fat exchange	Sodium	42 mg
	Potassium	261 mg
	Calories	66

Chocolate Almond Mocha Parfait

1 4-serving envelope D-zerta chocolate pudding mix
1¾ cups skim milk
1¼ oz envelope D'Zerta whip topping mix
2 tsp instant coffee powder
¼ cup slivered almonds

1. In saucepan, combine pudding mix and skim milk.

2. Cook and stir until mixture boils. Remove from heat. Cool.

3. Prepare topping according to package directions.

4. Combine topping mix and instant coffee powder.

5. Alternately spoon pudding and topping into 4 parfait glasses.

6. Top with almonds.

7. Chill.

Yield: 4 servings

1 serving: ½ skim milk exchange	Protein	5 gm
1 fat exchange	Fat	4 gm
½ fruit exchange	Carbohydrate	11 gm
	Sodium	119 mg
	Potassium	227 mg
	Calories	81

Chocolate Fondue

1 tbsp butter
2 tbsp cocoa
1 tbsp cornstarch
1 pinch salt
1 cup skim milk
2 tsp sugar substitute
½ tsp vanilla

1. Melt butter.

2. Combine cocoa, cornstarch, and salt.

3. Blend with melted butter until smooth.

4. Add milk and sugar substitute and cook over moderate heat, stirring constantly until slightly thickened.

5. Remove from heat. Stir in vanilla.

6. Set pan in ice water and stir until cool.

Yield: 16 tbsp

1 tbsp: free food exchange	Protein	0.5 gm
	Fat	0.7 gm
	Carbohydrate	1 gm
	Sodium	22 mg
	Potassium	27 mg
	Calories	12
5 tbsp: 1 vegetable exchange ½ fat exchange	Protein	2.5 gm
	Fat	3.5 gm
	Carbohydrate	5 gm
	Sodium	110 mg
	Potassium	135 mg
	Calories	61

Chocolate Sauce

1 envelope D'zerta Chocolate pudding
1 cup skim milk
1 cup water
1 square semi-sweet chocolate
1 tsp vanilla or desired extract

1. Combine the pudding powder, milk, and water in the top of a double boiler and add semi-sweet chocolate to melt.

2. Bring mixture to a boil, stirring occasionally.

3. Remove from heat.

4. Add vanilla or desired extract.

5. Chill.

Yield: 2 cups (32 tbsp)

2 tbsp: free food exchange	Protein	0 gm
	Fat	0 gm
	Carbohydrate	3 gm
	Sodium	8 mg
	Potassium	28 mg
	Calories	12
¼ cup: ½ fruit exchange	Protein	1 gm
	Fat	1 gm
	Carbohydrate	6 gm
	Sodium	16 mg
	Potassium	56 mg
	Calories	37

Chocolate Bavarian

¾ tsp gelatin, unflavored
⅗ tbsp water
1½ tbsp cocoa
6 tbsp skim milk
¼ tbsp liquid artificial sweetener
⅛ tsp vanilla
6 tbsp non-fat skim milk powder
6 tbsp ice water

1. Soften the gelatin in the water.

2. Make a paste of the cocoa and fluid milk. Heat over boiling water.

3. Add softened gelatin and liquid artificial sweetener.

4. Stir until gelatin is dissolved.

5. Remove mixture from heat; cool until mixture thickens. Mixture thickens quickly.

6. Add vanilla.

7. Combine ice water and dry milk in bowl and beat until mixture has the consistency of whipped cream.

8. Beat gelatin mixture until smooth and gradually add to whipped milk.

9. Spoon onto oiled pan.

10. Chill until firm—about three hours. Chocolate Bavarian should be used same day it is made.

Yield: 5 servings
1 serving: ½ skim milk exchange

Protein	4 gm
Fat	0 gm
Carbohydrate	6 gm
Sodium	56 mg
Potassium	209 mg
Calories	40

Heavenly Ambrosia

1-6 oz package orange-flavored gelatin
2 cups boiling water
1¼ cups cold water
1 cup plain yogurt
1½ tsp grated orange peel
1 cup orange slices
1 cup grapefruit sections
1 banana, sliced
2 tbsp coconut

1. Dissolve gelatin in boiling water. Add cold water. Chill until almost set.

2. Add yogurt and orange peel. Whip with beater until blended.

3. Pour into 4½ cup mold.

4. Chill until firm.

5. Unmold on platter.

6. Serve with combined fruits and coconut.

Yield: 8 servings (4 cups)

½ cup: 2 bread-starch exchanges

Protein	4 gm
Fat	1 gm
Carbohydrate	29 gm
Sodium	84 mg
Potassium	180 mg
Calories	141

¼ cup: 1 bread-starch exchange

Protein	2 gm
Fat	0 gm
Carbohydrate	15 gm
Sodium	42 mg
Potassium	90 mg
Calories	68

Fruit Cocktail Mold

½ **envelope artificially sweetened flavored gelatin**
½ **cup boiling water**
½ **cup cold water**
1 **cup unsweetened fruit cocktail**

1. Drain fruit cocktail.

2. Dissolve gelatin in boiling water.

3. Add cold water.

4. Put in refrigerator to chill.

5. Measure ¼ cup fruit cocktail into four molds.

6. Pour gelatin over fruit.

7. Chill until set.

Yield: 4 servings (2 cups)
½ cup: 1 fruit exchange

Protein	0 gm
Fat	0 gm
Carbohydrate	6 gm
Sodium	3 mg
Potassium	103 mg
Calories	24

Apple Fluff

½ envelope lemon-flavored artificially sweetened gelatin
1 cup boiling water
1 cup applesauce, unsweetened
¼ tsp liquid artificial sweetener
¼ tsp cinnamon

1. Dissolve gelatin in boiling water.

2. Chill until set.

3. Mix cinnamon and liquid artificial sweetener into applesauce.

4. When gelatin is set, whip until thick and lemon-yellow in color.

5. Fold gelatin into applesauce mixture.

6. Pile into four individual sherbets and chill.

Yield: 4 servings
1 serving: ½ fruit exchange

Protein	9 gm
Fat	0 gm
Carbohydrate	6 gm
Sodium	1 mg
Potassium	47 mg
Calories	24

Apricot Dessert

1 cup unsweetened, drained apricots
½ cup apricot liquid
½ envelope lemon-flavored artificially sweetened gelatin
2 whole cloves
⅓ cup boiling water
1½ tsp lemon juice
½ tsp liquid artificial sweetener

1. Mash apricots or puree in blender.

2. Mix apricot liquid with gelatin, set aside.

3. Add cloves to boiling water.

4. Simmer 5 minutes.

5. Remove cloves.

6. Stir in softened gelatin until dissolved.

7. Add liquid artificial sweetener, salt, lemon juice and mashed apricots.

8. Pour into three molds.

9. Chill until firm.

10. Unmold.

Yield: 3 servings
⅔ cup: 1 fruit exchange

Protein	0 gm
Fat	0 gm
Carbohydrate	8 gm
Sodium	0 mg
Potassium	205 mg
Calories	32

Blueberry Dessert

½ cup drained, unsweetened canned blueberries
¼ tsp liquid artificial sweetener
½ tsp lemon juice
⅓ cup blueberry juice
½ envelope strawberry-flavored artificially sweetened gelatin
3 tbsp water

1. Heat blueberry juice and water to boiling.

2. Dissolve gelatin in liquid.

3. When gelatin is completely dissolved, add blueberries, lemon juice, and liquid artificial sweetener.

4. Mix to blend thoroughly.

5. Pour into three individual molds.

6. Chill until set.

Yield: 3 servings (1½ cups)
½ cup: ½ fruit exchange

Protein	1 gm
Fat	0 gm
Carbohydrate	7 gm
Sodium	7 mg
Potassium	49 mg
Calories	32

Lemon Froth With Blueberries

1 envelope lemon-flavored artificially sweetened gelatin
½ cup boiling water
½ cup artificially sweetened lemon-lime flavored pop or soft drink
2 tsp grated lemon peel
1⅓ cups fresh or unsweetened blueberries

1. Dissolve gelatin in boiling water.

2. Add cold pop or soft drink and lemon peel.

3. Chill.

4. Whip gelatin mixture.

5. Spoon into four dessert dishes and top with ⅓ cup blueberries.

Yield: 4 servings
1 serving: 1 fruit exchange

Protein	2 gm
Fat	0 gm
Carbohydrate	7 gm
Sodium	35 mg
Potassium	46 mg
Calories	36

Lemon Snow

1 tsp gelatin
1 tbsp cold water
½ cup hot water
½ tsp liquid artificial sweetener
1 tbsp lemon juice
1 egg white

1. Soften gelatin in cold water.

2. Mix together hot water, liquid artificial sweetener, and lemon juice.

3. Heat.

4. Dissolve gelatin in hot water mixture.

5. Chill until set.

6. Beat egg white until stiff.

7. Fold into gelatin mixture which has been whipped.

8. Pile into two sherbet glasses.

Yield: 2 servings
1 serving: free food exchange

Protein	4 gm
Fat	0 gm
Carbohydrate	1 gm
Sodium	27 mg
Potassium	47 mg
Calories	20

Orange Fluff

½ envelope lemon-flavored artificially sweetened gelatin
½ cup orange juice
½ cup hot water
½ cup unsweetened mandarin oranges

First stage

1. Combine orange juice and water.

2. Heat to boiling.

3. Dissolve lemon gelatin in this boiling mixture.

4. Chill overnight.

Second stage

5. Whip gelatin mixture.

6. Fold in oranges.

7. Pile into two sherbet glasses.

Yield: 2 servings
1 serving: 1 fruit exchange

Protein	2 gm
Fat	0 gm
Carbohydrate	12 gm
Sodium	11 mg
Potassium	214 mg
Calories	56

Peach Whip

2¼ tsp plain gelatin
⅜ tsp liquid artificial sweetener
⅛ tsp salt
2 cups less 3 tbsp water
¼ cup concentrated frozen orange juice
3 egg whites
1 cup pureed unsweetened peaches
⅛ tsp almond flavoring

1. Mix gelatin, liquid artificial sweetener, salt, and a small amount of water.

2. Place over low heat.

3. Stir constantly until the gelatin dissolves.

4. Remove from heat.

5. Add remaining water and juice.

6. Chill until slightly thicker than unbeaten egg white consistency.

7. Fold in beaten egg whites and pureed peaches and almond flavoring.

8. Chill until firm.

Yield: 6 servings
1 serving: 1½ fruit exchange

OR

1 bread-starch
exchange

Protein	3 gm
Fat	0 gm
Carbohydrate	14 gm
Sodium	72 mg
Potassium	258 mg
Calories	68

Pineapple Fluff

1 slice drained unsweetened pineapple
½ tsp lemon juice
3 tbsp unsweetened pineapple juice
¼ tsp liquid artificial sweetener
½ envelope lemon-flavored artificially sweetened gelatin
1 egg white

1. Puree pineapple in blender or chop fine.

2. Heat pineapple juice to boiling.

3. Dissolve gelatin in the liquid.

4. When gelatin is completely dissolved, add liquid artificial sweetener, lemon juice and pureed pineapple. Mix well.

5. Chill to unbeaten egg white consistency.

6. Fold in egg white, stiffly beaten.

7. Pile into three individual sherbets.

8. Chill until firm.

Yield: 3 servings
1 serving: ½ fruit exchange

Protein	1 gm
Fat	0 gm
Carbohydrate	6 gm
Sodium	19 mg
Potassium	83 mg
Calories	28

Strawberry Sponge

1 tbsp unflavored gelatin
½ cup cold water
1⅓ tbsp liquid artificial sweetener
1 tbsp lemon juice
1 cup strawberries, crushed
2 egg whites

1. Soften gelatin in water in top half of a double boiler.

2. Add liquid artificial sweetener and lemon juice.

3. Stir until gelatin dissolves.

4. Remove from heat.

5. Add the crushed strawberries

6. Let stand until mixture begins to thicken.

7. Beat until light and fluffy.

8. Beat egg whites and fold into the mixture.

9. Chill until firm. May garnish with fresh strawberry.

Yield: 3 servings

1 serving: ½ skim milk exchange	Protein	6 gm
OR	Fat	0 gm
	Carbohydrate	4 gm
½ fruit exchange	Sodium	37 mg
1 meat, medium fat exchange	Potassium	123 mg
add 1 fat exchange to your meal plan	Calories	40

Popsicles

½ cup orange juice or ¼ cup grape juice
1 tsp lemon juice
¼ tsp liquid artificial sweetener

1. Combine ingredients.

2. Pour into a mold.

3. Freeze.

Yield: 1 serving
1 serving: 1 fruit exchange

1 orange popsicle:		
Protein	1 gm
Fat	0 gm
Carbohydrate	13 gm
Sodium	1 mg
Potassium	225 mg
Calories	56

1 grape popsicle:		
Protein	0 gm
Fat	0 gm
Carbohydrate	10 gm
Sodium	1 mg
Potassium	82 mg
Calories	40

Foamy Sauce

2 egg whites
2 egg yolks
1 cup sifted powdered sugar
½ cup whipping cream
¼ tsp vanilla

1. In large bowl, beat egg whites to stiff peaks, gradually adding sifted powdered sugar.

2. Beat egg yolks and vanilla until thick.

3. Fold into egg whites.

4. In small bowl whip whipping cream until soft peaks form.

5. Fold whipped cream mixture into egg mixture.

Yield: 2 cups (32 tbsp)
1 tbsp: ½ fruit exchange

Protein	0 gm
Fat	1 gm
Carbohydrate	4 gm
Sodium	5 mg
Potassium	9 mg
Calories	29

Fruit Soup

½ cup tapioca
1 cup raisins
1 cup prunes
1 stick of cinnamon
4 cups hot water
2 cups canned peaches, diced
  (water or juice packed)
1 cup raspberry juice or grape juice
2 tbsp vinegar
½ cup sugar

1. Add first 4 ingredients to water and boil until tapioca is transparent.

2. Simmer slowly until raisins and prunes are tender.

3. Add peaches, juice, lemon juice, and sugar.

4. Serve hot or cold.

Yield: 4 cups
¼ cup: 3 fruit exchanges

Protein	2.6 gm
Fat	0 gm
Carbohydrate	30 gm
Sodium	5 mg
Potassium	211 mg
Calories	130

East Indian Fruit Compote

1⅔ cups unsweetened pineapple tidbits, drained
1 cup red apple slices, unpared
1 cup orange sections, drained
1 cup grapefruit sections, drained
½ cup sour cream
½ tsp curry powder
¼ tsp salt
¼ tsp liquid artificial sweetener

1. Combine fruit.

2. Blend remaining ingredients.

3. Serve over fruit.

Yield: 6 servings
1 serving: 1 vegetable exchange
         1 fruit exchange
         1 fat exchange

Protein	1 gm
Fat	5 gm
Carbohydrate	18 gm
Sodium	99 mg
Potassium	321 mg
Calories	121

Ambrosia

1½ cups unsweetened pineapple chunks, drained
3 oranges, peeled and cut into chunks
1 tbsp coconut flakes

1. Combine fruits.

2. Just before serving, sprinkle coconut on top of fruits.

Yield: 6 servings
1 serving: 1 fruit exchange

Protein	1 gm
Fat	0 gm
Carbohydrate	13 gm
Sodium	1 mg
Potassium	190 mg
Calories	56

Fruit Cup

1 banana, medium
1 raw apple
¼ melon
peaches, ½ cup (water or juice packed), drained
1 cup blueberries
3 tbsp frozen orange concentrate
2 tbsp pina colada drink mix

1. Cut, chip, and dice fruit.

2. Add juice and mix. Toss.

3. Refrigerate.

Yield: 2 cups

½ cup: 2 fruit exchanges		
Protein	1 gm
Fat	0 gm
Carbohydrate	22 gm
Sodium	5 mg
Potassium	349 mg
Calories	92

¼ cup: 1 fruit exchange		
Protein	0 gm
Fat	0 gm
Carbohydrate	11 gm
Sodium	4 mg
Potassium	174 mg
Calories	44

Orange and Apple Cocktail

1 small orange
1 small apple
¼ cup lemon juice
¼ cup water

1. Peel and dice both orange and apple.

2. Combine lemon juice and water.

3. Pour over fruit.

4. Mix well.

5. Chill.

6. Serve.

Yield: 2 servings
1 serving: 1 fruit exchange

Protein	1 gm
Fat	0 gm
Carbohydrate	13 gm
Sodium	1 mg
Potassium	232 mg
Calories	56

Peach Float

4 egg whites
6 peaches

1. Take the whites of four eggs, beat to a stiff froth.

2. Stew six peaches until soft enough to mash.

3. Beat in the whites of the eggs.

4. Dish into six servings.

5. Chill.

Yield: 6 servings
1 serving: 1 fruit exchange

Protein	3 gm
Fat	0 gm
Carbohydrate	13 gm
Sodium	38 mg
Potassium	304 mg
Calories	64

Baked Apples

1 small apple
dash of cinnamon and/or nutmeg
¼ tsp liquid artificial sweetener

1. Core apple and place in baking dish.

2. Sprinkle with cinnamon and/or nutmeg.

3. Add liquid artificial sweetener.

4. Cover tightly so that juices will not evaporate.

5. Bake in moderate oven (375 degrees) for 45–60 minutes.

Yield: 1 serving
1 serving: 1½ fruit exchanges

Protein	0 gm
Fat	0 gm
Carbohydrate	15 gm
Sodium	1 mg
Potassium	116 mg
Calories	60

Mint Pear

1 pear, ripe
6 mint leaf springs
1 cup strawberries

1. Wash and cut pear in half.

2. Wash and chop mint leaves.

3. Roll each pear half in the mint leaves.

4. Placing a lettuce leaf on a dish, set a pear half on it and then fill the center with ½ cup of strawberries, allowing the extra ones to be placed on the sides of the pear.

5. Chill and serve.

Yield: 2 servings
1 serving: 1 fruit exchange

Protein	0 gm
Fat	0 gm
Carbohydrate	12 gm
Sodium	1 mg
Potassium	175 mg
Calories	48

Prune Whip

3 dried prunes
⅔ tsp lemon juice
⅓ tsp liquid artificial sweetener
½ cup artificially sweetened commercial whipped topping

1. Cover prunes with water.

2. Cook until very well done. Remove pits.

3. Puree in blender or mash well with some of the liquid.

4. Mix with lemon juice and artificial sweetener.

5. Fold in whipped topping.

6. Divide into two sherbet glasses.

Yield: 2 servings
1 serving: 1 fruit exchange
          1 fat exchange

Protein	0 gm
Fat	4 gm
Carbohydrate	11 gm
Sodium	21 mg
Potassium	122 mg
Calories	60

Pie Crust

2 cups flour
1 tsp salt
¾ cup lard
¼ cup water
1 egg
1 tbsp vinegar

1. Mix flour, salt, and lard until crumbly with a fork.

2. Add water, egg, and vinegar. Blend. Knead slightly.

3. Divide into 4 parts. Roll into pie shape.

4. Bake according to filling used.

Yield: four 1 crust pies or two 2
      crust pies

⅙ of a 2 crust pie:	1 bread-starch exchange	Protein	3 gm
	3 fat exchanges	Fat	14 gm
		Carbohydrate	17 gm
		Sodium	184 mg
		Potassium	28 mg
		Calories	206
⅙ of a 1 crust pie:	1 fruit exchange	Protein	1 gm
	1 fat exchange	Fat	7 gm
		Carbohydrate	9 gm
		Sodium	92 mg
		Potassium	14 mg
		Calories	103

Graham Cracker Crust

2 tbsp margarine
2 tbsp warm water
3 tbsp sugar
12 graham crackers (large rectangles, crumbled)

1. Melt margarine.

2. Add water and sugar.

3. Stir in graham crackers.

4. Bake at 400 degrees for 6–8 minutes.

5. Cool.

Yield: 8 servings

⅛ pie:	1 bread-starch exchange		
	½ fruit exchange	Protein	2 gm
	1 fat exchange	Fat	5 gm
		Carbohydrate	20 gm
		Sodium	177 mg
		Potassium	83 mg
		Calories	133

Crumb Crust

3 tbsp margarine
1 tbsp sugar
¾ cup cornflake crumbs (2¼ cups cornflakes)

1. Heat oven to 375 degrees.

2. In a 9-inch pie plate, mix together margarine, sugar, and cornflake crumbs.

3. When mixture is crumbly, press mixture with back of a spoon into bottom and up the sides of the pie plate. Crust will be thin.

4. Bake 8 minutes.

5. Cool. Fill with your choice of filling.

Yield: 1 (9-inch) crumb crust

⅙ of crust: 1 fruit exchange 1 fat exchange		
	Protein	1 gm
	Fat	6 gm
	Carbohydrate	11 gm
	Sodium	174 mg
	Potassium	14 mg
	Calories	102

⅛ of crust: ¾ fruit exchange 1 fat exchange		
	Protein	0.6 gm
	Fat	4 gm
	Carbohydrate	8 gm
	Sodium	130 mg
	Potassium	11 mg
	Calories	70

1/10 of crust: ½ fruit exchange ½ fat exchange		
	Protein	0.5 gm
	Fat	3 gm
	Carbohydrate	7 gm
	Sodium	104 mg
	Potassium	8 mg
	Calories	57

"Old Fashioned" Pumpkin Pie

chilled uncooked pastry shell, 9 inch
3 eggs
1 tsp pumpkin pie spice
1 tbsp liquid artificial sweetener
2 tbsp melted butter or margarine
1½ cups cooked hot pumpkin
1½ cups scalded skim milk

1. Beat eggs.

2. Add, in order, spices, salt, sweetener, melted shortening, hot pumpkin, and scalded skim milk.

3. Pour into pastry shell.

4. Bake at 450 degrees for 10 minutes.

Yield: 9 or 12 servings

⅑ pie:	2 bread-starch exchanges		
	2 fat exchanges	Protein	5 gm
		Fat	11 gm
		Carbohydrate	32 gm
		Sodium	195 mg
		Potassium	285 mg
		Calories	247
¹⁄₁₂ pie:	1 bread-starch exchange		
	1 fruit exchange	Protein	4 gm
	1½ fat exchanges	Fat	8 gm
		Carbohydrate	24 gm
		Sodium	146 mg
		Potassium	214 mg
		Calories	184

Yam Peanut Pie

3 eggs
¾ cup sugar
1 cup yams, mashed
1½ tbsp margarine
½ cup light corn syrup
1½ tbsp flour
a few grains of salt
1 tsp cinnamon
¼ tsp mace
½ tsp vanilla
⅔ cup chopped salted peanuts
1-9 inch unbaked pie shell

1. Beat eggs slightly with a fork.

2. Add sugar, yams, margarine, and syrup to eggs.

3. Stir in flour, salt, cinnamon, mace, and vanilla.

4. Add ½ cup peanuts.

5. Pour into pie shell.

6. Bake at 350 degrees for 30 minutes.

7. Remove from oven. Sprinkle remaining peanuts over top.

8. Return to oven for 30 minutes.

Yield: 12 pieces

1/12 pie: 1½ bread-starch
        exchanges
      2 fat exchanges

Protein	5 gm
Fat	11 gm
Carbohydrate	22 gm
Sodium	168 mg
Potassium	126 mg
Calories	207

Pumpkin Chiffon Pie

1 tbsp (1 envelope) unflavored gelatin
½ cup cold water
2 eggs, separated
1 cup canned or cooked pumpkin
⅓ cup sugar
1 tsp vanilla
½ tsp cinnamon
¼ tsp salt
¼ tsp nutmeg
⅓ cup instant skim milk powder
⅓ cup ice water
¾ cup graham cracker crumbs
2 tbsp butter

1. Melt butter.

2. Mix into graham cracker crumbs. Press into pie plate.

3. Chill.

4. Chill small mixer bowl and beaters in refrigerator.

5. In medium saucepan, soften gelatin in cold water.

6. Heat over medium heat until gelatin dissolves.

7. Add egg yolks, pumpkin, sugar, vanilla, cinnamon, salt, and nutmeg. Stir.

8. In small chilled mixer bowl, beat skim milk powder, ice water, and egg whites at high speed until stiff peaks form.

9. Fold into pumpkin mixture.

10. Carefully pour into chilled pie shell.

11. Chill about 2 hours or until firm.

Yield: 8 servings

⅛ of pie:	1 bread-starch exchange	Protein	4 gm
	1 vegetable exchange	Fat	5 gm
	1 fat exchange	Carbohydrate	19 gm
		Sodium	198 mg
		Potassium	203 mg
		Calories	137

(continued)

Pumpkin Chiffon Pie (continued)

OR

Yield: 6 servings

⅙ of pie: 1 bread-starch exchange
1½ fat exchanges
1 vegetable exchange

Protein	6 gm
Fat	7 gm
Carbohydrate	25 gm
Sodium	264 mg
Potassium	270 mg
Calories	187

Pumpkin Dessert

16 oz pumpkin
1½ tbsp artificial brown sugar
½ tsp salt
½ tsp cinnamon
½ tsp nutmeg
½ tsp butter flavoring
8 oz evaporated skim milk

---

1. Combine ingredients.

2. Pour into 8-inch pie pan without a crust.

3. Bake 20 minutes at 450 degrees then at 350 degrees until done. (A knife should come out clean.)

Yield: 6 pieces

1 serving: 1 fruit exchange
½ meat, medium fat exchange
you can add ½ fat exchange to your meal

Protein	4 gm
Fat	0 gm
Carbohydrate	10 gm
Sodium	312 mg
Potassium	309 mg
Calories	56

Pumpkin Parfait Pie

1 envelope unflavored gelatin
1½ cup skim milk
1 cup canned pumpkin
½ tsp cinnamon
¼ tsp nutmeg
¼ tsp ginger
⅛ tsp cloves
1 cup vanilla ice cream, softened
⅓ cup sugar
½ tsp vanilla
3 drops red food coloring
2 drops yellow food coloring
graham cracker crust

1. In a saucepan soften gelatin in skim milk.

2. Blend in pumpkin and spices.

3. Cook over low heat, stirring constantly, until it comes to a boil.

4. Remove from heat.

5. Blend in remaining ingredients until well combined.

6. Chill until slightly thickened but not set.

7. By hand, stir briskly until smooth and pour into graham cracker crumb crust.

8. Chill until firm for about 2 to 3 hours.

Yield: 6 or 9 servings

⅙ pie: 3 bread-starch exchanges 1½ fat exchanges		
Protein	5 gm
Fat	8 gm
Carbohydrate	48 gm
Sodium	282 mg
Potassium	330 mg
Calories	284

⅑ pie: 2 bread-starch exchanges 1 fat exchange		
Protein	4 gm
Fat	5 gm
Carbohydrate	32 gm
Sodium	188 mg
Potassium	220 mg
Calories	189

(continued)

Pumpkin Parfait Pie (continued)

¹⁄₁₂ pie:	1 bread-starch exchange	Protein	3 gm
	1 fruit exchange	Fat	4 gm
	1 fat exchange	Carbohydrate	24 gm
		Sodium	141 mg
		Potassium	165 mg
		Calories	144

Frozen Pumpkin Pie

1 cup pumpkin, mashed and cooked
½ cup dark corn syrup
½ tsp salt
½ tsp ginger
¼ tsp nutmeg
¼ tsp cinnamon
1 cup heavy cream
¼ cup sugar
1 pint vanilla ice cream, softened
baked graham crust

1. Mix first 6 ingredients.

2. Whip cream. Beat in sugar. Fold into pumpkin mixture.

3. Spread ice cream on crust.

4. Spoon pumpkin mixture over the ice cream.

5. Freeze for at least 2 hours.

Yield: 12 servings

1 serving:	2 bread-starch exchanges	Protein	3 gm
		Fat	13 gm
	½ fruit exchange	Carbohydrate	34 gm
	2½ fat exchanges	Sodium	269 mg
		Potassium	159 mg
	OR	Calories	265
	1 bread-starch exchange		
	2 fruit exchanges		
	2½ fat exchanges		

Cranberry Mince Pie

1 cup granulated sugar substitute
½ tsp salt
½ tsp cloves
½ tsp ginger
1 tsp cinnamon
1⅓ cups seedless raisins
⅓ cup chopped walnuts
1 tbsp grated orange peel
2 tsp grated lemon peel
⅓ cup lemon juice
¾ cup jellied cranberry sauce (artificially sweetened)
1⅓ cups finely chopped apple
your favorite pie crust recipe

1. Combine the sugar substitute, salt, and spices.

2. Add raisins, nuts, peels, lemon juice, cranberry sauce, and apple. Mix well.

3. Pour into pie crust.

4. Bake in hot oven at 400 degrees for about 35 minutes.

⅛ pie:	1 fruit exchange	Protein	9 gm
	2 bread-starch exchanges	Fat	11 gm
	2 fat exchanges	Carbohydrate	37 gm
		Sodium	340 mg
		Potassium	290 mg
		Calories	283

1/12 pie:	1 bread-starch exchange	Protein	6 gm
	1 fruit exchange	Fat	7 gm
	1 fat exchange	Carbohydrate	25 gm
	OR	Sodium	227 mg
		Potassium	193 mg
	2½ fruit exchanges	Calories	187
	1 meat low-fat exchange		
	1 fat exchange		

Lime-Chiffon Pie

20 small chocolate wafer cookies
1 package low calorie lime-flavored gelatin
1 cup boiling water
3 oz (½ small can) frozen limeade
½ cup cold water
1 tbsp lime juice
1 cup evaporated skim milk
2 drops green food coloring, if desired

1. Line 9-inch lightly oiled pie tin with chocolate wafer crumbs.

2. Dissolve lime gelatin in boiling water. Add frozen limeade and cold water.

3. Chill until partially set.

4. Chill milk, bowl, and beaters several hours before whipping. Whip evaporated skim milk.

5. Fold whipped skim milk into partially set gelatin.

6. Add lime juice and green coloring.

7. Put into crumb-lined pan and chill until set.

8. Serve with low calorie whipped topping.

Yield: 6 servings

⅙ pie: 2 bread-starch exchanges		
1 fat exchange	Protein	4 gm
½ fruit exchange	Fat	6 gm
1 tbsp whipped topping: free food exchange	Carbohydrate	35 gm
	Sodium	106 mg
	Potassium	159 mg
	Calories	210

Homemade Mincemeat Pie

1 lb beef stew meat
4 lb apples
4 oz suet
1-15 oz package of raisins
2½ cups sugar
2½ cups water
2 cups dried currants
½ cup chopped mixed candied fruits and peels
1 tsp grated orange peel
1 cup orange juice
1 tsp grated lemon peel
¼ cup lemon juice
1 tsp salt
½ tsp ground nutmeg
¼ tsp ground mace
pastry for 2-crust 9-inch pie

1. Cover beef with water. Simmer covered until tender, about 2 hours.

2. Drain and cool.

3. Peel, core, and cut up apples.

4. Put beef, apples, and suet through coarse blade of food grinder.

5. In kettle combine all ingredients except pastry.

6. Cover. Simmer 1 hour. Stir often.

7. Line 9-inch pie plate with pastry.

8. Fill with 3 cups of mincemeat.

9. Adjust top crust. Seal. Cut slits.

10. Bake at 400 degrees for 35 to 40 minutes. Freeze remaining mincemeat in 3-cup portions. Makes 12 cups.

Food Exchange: one mincemeat pie (2 pie crusts and 3 cups mincemeat)

⅑ of pie:	2 bread-starch exchanges	Protein	5 gm
	2½ fruit exchanges	Fat	17 gm
	3 fat exchanges	Carbohydrate	54 gm
		Sodium	216 mg
		Potassium	272 mg
		Calories	389

(continued)

Homemade Mincemeat Pie (continued)

⅟₁₈ of pie:	1 bread-starch exchange 1 fruit exchange 1½ fat exchange	Protein	2 gm
		Fat	8 gm
		Carbohydrate	27 gm
		Sodium	158 mg
		Potassium	136 mg
		Calories	188

Minnesota Harvest Bars

¼ cup shortening
1 cup brown sugar
⅔ can of canned pumpkin
2 eggs
½ tsp vanilla
½ cup flour
½ tsp baking powder
½ tsp salt
½ tsp baking soda
½ tsp cinnamon
½ tsp nutmeg
½ tsp ginger
½ cup dates, chopped
½ cup walnuts, chopped, with 2 tbsp flour
⅛ cup powdered sugar

1. Melt shortening, add brown sugar and stir. Remove from heat.

2. Add pumpkin.

3. Add the remaining ingredients and mix.

4. Pour in greased pan, 13 x 9 x 2 inches.

5. Bake at 350 degrees for 30–35 minutes.

6. While warm, sift with powdered sugar.

Yield: 52-1½ inch squares

1 serving:	½ fruit exchange ½ fat exchange	Protein	0.7 gm
		Fat	2 gm
		Carbohydrate	6 gm
		Sodium	38 mg
		Potassium	44 mg
		Calories	45

Autumn Torte

½ cup butter
2 cups sugar
2 eggs, beaten
1 tsp soda
½ tsp baking powder
1 tsp cinnamon
1½ tsp salt
2 cups flour
1 cup nuts, chopped
6 cups apples (peeled and chopped)

1. Cream butter and sugar.

2. Add eggs.

3. Sift dry ingredients and add to creamed mixture.

4. Stir in nuts and apples.

5. Spread in 9 x 13 inch greased and floured pan.

6. Bake at 350 degrees for 40–45 minutes.

7. Serve with 1 tbsp dream whip.

Yield: 15 or 30 servings

⅟₁₅ serving:	2 bread-starch exchanges	Protein	5 gm
	3 fruit exchanges	Fat	13 gm
	2½ fat exchanges	Carbohydrate	64 gm
	1 tbsp Dream Whip:	Sodium	360 mg
	free food exchange	Potassium	212 mg
		Calories	393
⅟₃₀ serving:	1 bread-starch exchange	Protein	2 gm
	1½ fruit exchanges	Fat	6 gm
	1 fat exchange	Carbohydrate	32 gm
		Sodium	180 mg
		Potassium	106 mg
		Calories	190

Apple Crisp

4 cups apples (4 apples)
1 tbsp liquid artificial sweetener
1 tbsp lemon juice
1 tbsp cinnamon
2 tbsp butter (melted)
½ cup graham crackers, crushed (6 squares)
2 slices bread crumbs
½ tsp liquid artificial sweetener

1. Pare and slice apples.

2. Place in a 1½ quart casserole.

3. Sprinkle with artificial sweetener, lemon juice and cinnamon.

4. Combine butter, graham cracker crumbs, bread crumbs, and artificial sweetener.

5. Toss with fork until well combined.

6. Sprinkle over apples.

7. Pour ¾ cup hot water over topping.

8. Cover.

9. Bake at 400 degrees for 15 minutes.

10. Uncover and bake 15 to 20 minutes.

11. Serve warm.

Yield: 4 servings

1 serving:	1 bread-starch exchange	Protein	2 gm
	1½ fruit exchanges	Fat	7 gm
	1½ fat exchanges	Carbohydrate	30 gm
		Sodium	208 mg
		Potassium	246 mg
		Calories	191

Danish Puff or Swedish Kringle

Crust

1 cup flour
½ cup margarine
2 tbsp water

Filling

1 cup flour
1 cup water
½ cup margarine
3 eggs
1 tsp almond extract

Frosting

1 cup confectioner's sugar
water to thin
½ cup chopped nuts

Crust

1. Mix ingredients as for a pie crust.

2. Divide dough in half.

3. Pat each half with hands into strips.

4. Place about 3 inches apart on cookie sheet.

Filling

1. Melt margarine in water and bring to rolling boil. Add flavoring.

2. Remove from heat and immediately add flour and mix.

3. Add 1 egg at a time beating until smooth.

4. Spread half of mixture on each crust.

5. Bake at 400 degrees for 20 minutes then reduce to 350 degrees until brown and crisp. Total baking time is about 50 or 60 minutes.

6. Frost with icing and sprinkle with chopped nuts.

(continued)

Danish Puff or Swedish Kringle (continued)

Yield: 26 (1″ wide, 3″ long)

1 serving: 1 bread-starch exchange 2 fat exchanges	Protein	2 gm
	Fat	11 gm
	Carbohydrate	13 gm
	Sodium	93 mg
	Potassium	31 mg
	Calories	159

Strawberry Shortcake

1 cup strawberries
1 2-inch diameter baking powder biscuit
1 tbsp heavy cream

1. Split the biscuit.

2. Slice the strawberries.

3. Place ½ of the strawberries on the bottom half of the biscuit.

4. Place the top half of the biscuit on top.

5. Cover with remaining strawberries.

6. Beat the cream and top the dessert.

Yield: 1 serving

1 serving: 1 bread-starch exchange 1 fruit exchange 1 fat exchange	Protein	3 gm
	Fat	6 gm
	Carbohydrate	27 gm
	Sodium	138 mg
	Potassium	291 mg
	Calories	174

Date Roll

1 lb dates
2 cups bisquick
⅔ cup milk

Icing

½ cup powdered sugar
1–2 tsp milk
¼ cup chopped nuts

1. Chop dates.

2. Add water to cover dates.

3. Boil until soft and water is gone.

4. Cool.

5. Add milk to bisquick.

6. Knead until firm, about 10 minutes.

7. Divide in half.

8. Roll out each half.

9. Spread date filling on each half.

10. Roll up like a jelly roll.

11. Bake at 400 degrees until brown. Cool.

12. Mix icing.

13. Spread on rolls.

Yield: 2 rolls—8 or 16 slices per roll.

⅛ serving:		
1 bread-starch exchange	Protein	2 gm
2 fruit exchanges	Fat	4 gm
1 fat exchange	Carbohydrate	35 gm
	Sodium	200 mg
	Potassium	216 mg
	Calories	184

¹⁄₁₆ serving:		
1 bread-starch exchange	Protein	1 gm
½ fat exchange	Fat	2 gm
	Carbohydrate	17 gm
OR	Sodium	100 mg
	Potassium	108 mg
1½ fruit exchanges	Calories	90
½ fat exchange		

Eleanor's Deep Dark Secret

Cake

1 lb dates, cut up
1 cup walnuts, chopped
4 eggs
½ cup flour, sifted
1 tsp baking powder
¼ tsp salt
2 tsp vanilla

Topping

3 bananas (large)
2 oranges, cut up
1 cup crushed pineapple, unsweetened
1 cup whipping cream, whipped
6 cherries, cut in half
½ cup nuts, chopped

1. Mix ingredients for the cake in the order given. Sift flour, baking powder, and salt together before adding. Beat egg whites stiff and fold in last.

2. Spread in 9 x 13 inch pan.

3. Bake at 350 degrees for 30 minutes.

4. One hour before serving, break half of the cake in pieces and arrange on platter.

5. Arrange bananas and oranges over the cut-up cake.

6. Break the other half of the cake and pile on top of the fruit in a mound.

7. Pour the crushed pineapple over this.

8. Let stand until ready to use.

Before serving, spread whipping cream on top. Add nuts and cherries.

(continued)

Eleanor's Deep Dark Secret (continued)

Yield: 16 servings
      32 servings

1/16:	2 bread-starch exchanges		
	1/2 fruit exchange	Protein	5 gm
	2 fat exchanges	Fat	11 gm
		Carbohydrate	35 gm
		Sodium	70 mg
		Potassium	400 mg
		Calories	259

1/32:	1 bread-starch exchange		
	1 fat exchange	Protein	3 gm
		Fat	5 gm
		Carbohydrate	17 gm
		Sodium	35 mg
		Potassium	200 mg
		Calories	125

Fudge Cookies

2 tbsp butter
1½ cup chocolate chips
1 can Eagle Brand condensed milk
1 cup flour
1 tsp vanilla
½ cup nuts, ground

1. Melt butter, chocolate chips, and milk.

2. Cool until lukewarm.

3. Add flour, vanilla, and nuts.

4. Drop with a teaspoon onto a greased cookie sheet.

5. Bake at 350 degrees for 25 minutes.

Yield: 30 cookies

1 cookie:	1 bread-starch exchange		
	1 fat exchange	Protein	2 gm
		Fat	7 gm
		Carbohydrate	18 gm
		Sodium	27 mg
		Potassium	99 mg
		Calories	143

Pineapple Cheese Cake

Crust

1 cup Bran Chex or bran cereal
1 slice whole wheat bread
1 tbsp margarine

Filling

1 envelope gelatin
1-16 oz can crushed pineapple & juice (packed in its own juice)
1 tbsp lemon juice
1 cup cottage cheese
1 cup plain yogurt (low fat)
1 cup ricotta cheese
1 tbsp sugar

Crust

1. Blend cereal and bread until they form fine crumbs.

2. Mix margarine into mixture adding 3–4 tbsp of water.

3. Form in 9 inch pie tin.

4. Bake 10–12 minutes at 350 degrees.

Filling

5. Combine gelatin, pineapple juice, and lemon juice.

6. Heat until gelatin is dissolved.

7. Puree pineapple saving some crushed pineapple for garnish.

8. Blend cottage cheese until creamy.

9. Add yogurt and ricotta. Blend.

10. Add gelatin mixture, sugar, and pureed pineapple.

11. Pour into pie crust.

12. Chill 2–3 hours.

13. Garnish with saved crushed pineapple.

(continued)

Pineapple Cheese Cake (continued)

Yield: 9 servings

1 serving: 1 bread-starch exchange	Protein	9 gm
1 meat, low-fat exchange	Fat	3 gm
	Carbohydrate	15 gm
	Sodium	182 mg
	Potassium	169 mg
	Calories	123

Berliner Kranser

4 hard cooked egg yolks, mashed
4 raw egg yolks
1 lb butter or margarine
5 cups flour
1 cup sugar
1 tsp almond flavoring

---

1. Knead flour into butter.

2. Work the mashed boiled egg yolks together with raw egg yolks.

3. Add sugar and almond flavoring. Mix together well.

4. Form into wreaths.

5. Dip in slightly beaten egg white.

6. Bake at 350 degrees until light brown.

7. Add food coloring for variety.

Yield: 6 (72) dozen cookies

2 cookies: ½ fruit exchange	Protein	2 gm
1 bread-starch exchange	Fat	12 gm
2 fat exchanges	Carbohydrate	20 gm
	Sodium	126 mg
	Potassium	24 mg
	Calories	196
one cookie: 1 fruit exchange	Protein	1 gm
1 fat exchange	Fat	6 gm
	Carbohydrate	10 gm
	Sodium	63 mg
	Potassium	12 mg
	Calories	98

Lucious Cheesecake

2 tbsp butter or margarine, melted
⅓ cup corn-flake crumbs (using 1 cup of cornflakes)
¼ tsp granulated artificial sweetener
2 envelopes unflavored gelatin
1 tbsp liquid artificial sweetener
1 cup unsweetened orange juice
1 tsp lemon peel
2 tbsp lemon juice
2-8 oz containers of creamed cottage cheese
¾ cup heavy cream
3 egg whites
¼ tsp salt
1½ tsp unflavored gelatin
¼ cup water
½ tsp liquid artificial sweetener
2 cups hulled, fresh strawberries, partially crushed, or 2 cups
   frozen unsweetened, whole strawberries, thawed then
   crushed slightly

1. Mix together melted butter or margarine, corn-flake crumbs, and liquid artificial sweetener. Press this mixture evenly over the bottom of an 8 x 8½ inch cake pan.

2. Bake at 425 degrees for 5 to 7 minutes or until crumb mixture begins to brown very slightly around edges.

3. Cool.

4. In saucepan, mix together 2 envelopes gelatin, artificial sweetener, orange juice, lemon peel, and juice. Let stand to soften gelatin.

5. Sieve cottage cheese.

6. Heat gelatin mixture until gelatin is dissolved then add sieved cottage cheese.

7. Beat until smooth.

8. Stir in heavy cream until smooth.

9. Refrigerate until mixture has consistency of soft pudding.

10. Beat egg whites with salt until stiff, but dry peaks do not form.

11. Gently fold gelatin mixture into beaten egg whites until smooth.

(continued)

Luscious Cheesecake (continued)

12. Turn into cooled crumb mixture.

13. Refrigerate until set.

Glaze

1. Mix 1½ tsp gelatin with ¼ cup water and artificial sweetener. Let stand 5 minutes then bring to a simmer until gelatin is dissolved.

2. Stir in crushed strawberries.

3. Pour over cake and gently spread to edges.

4. Cover tightly with saran wrap or foil.

5. Refrigerate until completely set or about 3 hours.

Yield: 9 servings

1 serving: 1½ meat, medium fat exchanges
1 fruit exchange
1 fat exchange

Protein	11 gm
Fat	12 gm
Carbohydrate	11 gm
Sodium	261 mg
Potassium	196 mg
Calories	196

Almond Bark Candy

2 lbs almond bark
2 cups Captain Crunch peanut butter cereal
2 cups Rice Krispies
2 cups mini-marshmallows
1 cup salted peanuts

---

1. Melt almond bark in double boiler. (Do *not* let water boil).

2. Pour over other ingredients.

3. Drop onto waxed paper.

4. Keep in cool place.

Yield: 4 dozen (48 pieces)

1 piece: 1 bread-starch exchange
½ fat exchange

Protein	1 gm
Fat	3 gm
Carbohydrate	18 gm
Sodium	76 mg
Potassium	47 mg
Calories	103

Poor Man's Fruitcake

1⅓ cup raisins
1 cup packed brown sugar
¼ cup lard
1½ cup all-purpose flour
½ tsp baking soda
½ tsp salt
½ tsp ground cinnamon
½ tsp ground cloves

1. Heat raisins, sugar, lard, and 1 cup of water until sugar dissolves and lard melts.

2. Cool.

3. Stir together flour, soda, salt, and spices.

4. Add to lard mixture. Beat smooth.

5. Pour into greased and floured 8½ x 4½ x 2½ inch loaf pan.

6. Bake at 350 degrees for 45–50 minutes.

7. Cool in pan.

8. Wrap. Store overnight.

Yield: 16-½ inch pieces, or,
      32-¼ inch pieces

½ inch piece: 2 bread-starch exchanges ½ fat exchange		
Protein	4 gm
Fat	3 gm
Carbohydrate	32 gm
Sodium	114 mg
Potassium	152 mg
Calories	171

¼ inch piece: 1 bread-starch exchange		
Protein	2 gm
Fat	1 gm
Carbohydrate	16 gm
Sodium	57 mg
Potassium	76 mg
Calories	81

Fruit Cake

8 oz pitted dates, chopped (1½ cups)
8 oz candied pineapple, chopped (1 cup)
8 oz candied cherries, quartered (1 cup)
8 oz raisins (1 cup)
4 oz candied lemon peel, chopped (½ cup)
1 cup broken walnuts
1 cup broken pecans
2 cups all-purpose flour
1 cup shortening
½ cup sugar
½ cup honey
5 eggs
1 tsp salt
1 tsp baking powder
1 tsp ground allspice
½ tsp ground nutmeg
½ tsp ground cloves
⅓ cup orange or grape juice
¼ cup wine, brandy, or fruit juice

1. Combine dates, pineapple, cherries, raisins, lemon peel, orange peel, walnuts, and pecans.

2. Toss with ¼ cup of the flour.

3. Cream shortening and sugar.

4. Stir in honey.

5. Add eggs, one at a time, beating well after each.

6. Combine remaining flour, salt, baking powder, and spices.

7. Add to creamed mixture alternately with ⅓ cup orange or grape juice.

8. Beat well.

9. Pour batter over floured fruits. Mix well.

10. Pour into two greased and floured 11x4x3 inch loaf pans.

11. Bake at 275 degrees until done, about 2 hours.

12. Cool.

13. Soak cheesecloth in wine, brandy, or fruit juice.

(continued)

Fruit Cake (continued)

14. Wrap fruitcakes in cheesecloth, then in foil.

15. Store in cool place 1 to 2 weeks. Makes two loaves.

Yield: 2 loaves
        Cut in ½ inch slice: 22 slices per loaf
        Cut in ¼ inch slice: 44 slices per loaf

½ inch slice: 2 bread-starch exchanges 2 fat exchanges		
	Protein	3 gm
	Fat	9 gm
	Carbohydrate	30 gm
	Sodium	64 mg
	Potassium	127 mg
	Calories	213

¼ inch slice: 1 bread-starch exchange 1 fat exchange		
	Protein	1 gm
	Fat	4 gm
	Carbohydrate	15 gm
	Sodium	23 mg
	Potassium	63 mg
	Calories	100

Ice Cream Balls

1 cup graham cracker crumbs (about 14 single crackers)
¼ cup peanut butter
1 tbsp cinnamon
2 tbsp granulated artificial sweetener
8 cups vanilla ice cream

1. Mix together graham crackers, peanut butter, cinnamon, and artificial sweetener.

2. Roll scoops (½ cup) of vanilla ice cream in the crumb mixture. May be served with dietetic chocolate sauce.

Yield: 16 balls

1 ice cream ball: 1 bread-starch exchange 2 fat exchanges		
	Protein	4 gm
	Fat	9 gm
	Carbohydrate	12 gm
	Sodium	102 mg
	Potassium	165 mg
	Calories	145

Potica Cake

Dough

1 cup margarine
½ cup milk
2 packages of yeast
¼ cup warm water
1 tsp warm water
1 tsp sugar
2½ cups flour
¼ tsp salt
2 tbsp sugar
3 egg yolks, beaten

Filling

½ cup walnuts, ground
3 tbsp sugar
¼ cup milk, warm
1 tsp cinnamon
½ cup dates, chopped
3 egg yolks, beaten
1 cup sugar

Dough

1. Melt margarine and milk. Cool.

2. Dissolve yeast and 1 tsp sugar in water.

3. Mix flour, salt and 2 tbsp sugar.

4. Add margarine and yeast mixture to flour mixture.

5. Make a hole in mixture.

6. Add egg yolks to mixture.

7. Refrigerate to cool.

Filling

8. Add sugar to 3 egg yolks.

9. Mix nuts, sugar, milk, cinnamon, and dates.

10. Add nut mixture to sugar mixture.

(continued)

Potica Cake (continued)

Cake Preparation

11. Roll dough out to an oblong piece that is paper thin.

12. Spread filling on dough.

13. Cut in half. Roll like a tube.

14. Put in angel food pan.

15. Bake at 350 degrees for 1 hour.

Yield: 30 slices, ¾ inch thick
1 slice: 1 bread-starch exchange
     ½ fruit exchange
     2 fat exchanges

Protein	2 gm
Fat	9 gm
Carbohydrate	20 gm
Sodium	97 mg
Potassium	51 mg
Calories	169

Rosettes

2 eggs
1 tsp sugar
¼ tsp salt
1 cup milk
1 cup flour
lard

1. Mix all ingredients together.

2. Dip rosette iron into batter being careful not to cover top of iron.

3. Fry in hot lard.

4. Drain rosettes upside down on paper towel.

Yield: 40
6 rosettes: ½ meat, medium-fat
     exchange
    1 bread-starch
     exchange
    1 fat exchange

Protein	5 gm
Fat	8 gm
Carbohydrate	18 gm
Sodium	117 mg
Potassium	91 mg
Calories	164

Easy Butter Cookies

4 cups flour
2 tsp baking powder
¼ tsp soda
½ tsp salt
1 cup butter or margarine (softened)
2 cups sugar
2 eggs
1½ tsp vanilla
¼ cup milk

1. Sift together flour, baking powder, soda, and salt.

2. In large mixing bowl, cream together butter, sugar, eggs, and flavoring.

3. Add milk.

4. Gradually stir in flour mixture, beating until blended.

5. Refrigerate dough until it is easy to handle.

6. Roll dough out thin on floured surface and cut with floured cutter. Lift with broad spatula onto greased cookie sheet.

7. Bake at 350 degrees for 12 minutes or until golden brown.

Yield: 24 dozen cookies
4 cookies: 1 fruit exchange
            ½ fat exchange

Protein	1 gm
Fat	3 gm
Carbohydrate	11 gm
Sodium	70 mg
Potassium	10 mg
Calories	75

Butter Cookies

½ lb unsalted butter (softened)
½ cup sugar
½ tsp vanilla
1½ cups flour
¼ tsp salt

1. Preheat oven to 350 degrees.

2. Cream butter, sugar, and vanilla until light and fluffy.

3. Combine flour and salt.

4. Sift into butter mixture ½ cup at a time beating well after each addition.

5. Scoop dough onto the center of a large ungreased baking sheet.

6. With meat spatula spread the dough into a 9-inch square pan about ½ inch thick.

7. Bake in middle of oven for about 35 minutes or until top is golden brown.

8. Remove pan from oven and cut into 1½ inch squares with a sharp knife.

9. Transfer the squares to a wire cake rack and when cool store in tightly covered container.

Yield: 3 dozen cookies
  (1½ inches square)
1 cookie: ½ bread-starch exchange
        1 fat exchange
2 cookies: 1 bread-starch exchange
        2 fat exchanges

1 cookie:		2 cookies:	
Protein	0.5 gm	Protein	1 gm
Fat	5 gm	Fat	10 gm
Carbohydrate	7 gm	Carbohydrate	14 gm
Sodium	16 mg	Sodium	32 mg
Potassium	5 mg	Potassium	10 mg
Calories	75	Calories	150

Crullers

⅓ **cup granulated sugar**
¼ **cup butter**
2 eggs
2 tbsp milk
½ **tsp salt**
½ **tsp ground nutmeg**
¼ **tsp ground mace**
fat for frying
powdered sugar

1. Cream together granulated sugar and butter until light and fluffy.

2. Add eggs, one at a time. Beat well after each addition.

3. Add milk (batter may appear slightly curdled).

4. Stir together flour, salt, nutmeg, and mace. Stir into the creamed mixture.

5. Chill at least one hour.

6. On lightly floured surface, roll half the dough (rolling in one direction only) to a 16 x 8 inch rectangle. Cut into 2 inch squares (do not reroll). Use a pastry wheel for pretty edges. Repeat with remaining dough.

7. Fry in deep hot fat (375 degrees) until golden on both sides, about 1½ minutes total.

8. Dust with powdered sugar.

Yield: 64 cookies
1 cookie: ½ fruit exchange
       1 fat exchange

Protein	0 gm
Fat	6 gm
Carbohydrate	5 gm
Sodium	27 mg
Potassium	3 mg
Calories	74

Thumb Print Cookies

½ cup butter
¼ cup brown sugar
1 egg yolk
1½ tsp vanilla
1 cup flour
¼ tsp salt
24 gum drops or 12 marachino cherries, halved

1. Cream butter. Add sugar gradually.

2. Blend in egg yolk and vanilla, mixing thoroughly.

3. Sift together flour and salt. Add gradually to mixture.

4. Shape into 24 small balls. Place on ungreased cookie sheet.

5. Bake at 350 degrees for 5 minutes.

6. Remove from oven. Press gum drop in center. Return to oven for 8–10 minutes.

Yield: 24 cookies

2 cookies:	1 bread-starch exchange		
	2 fat exchanges	Protein	2 gm
		Fat	8 gm
		Carbohydrate	14 gm
		Sodium	140 mg
		Potassium	24 mg
		Calories	136

Spritz

1½ cups butter or margarine
1 cup granulated sugar
1 egg
1 tsp vanilla
½ tsp almond extract
4 cups sifted all-purpose flour
1 tsp baking powder

1. Thoroughly cream butter and sugar.

2. Add egg, vanilla, and almond extract. Beat well.

3. Sift together flour and baking powder. Add gradually to creamed mixture, mixing to smooth dough. Do not chill.

4. Force dough through cookie press onto ungreased cookie sheet. Bake in hot oven (400 degrees) for 8 minutes. Cool.

Yield: 6 dozen (72) cookies

1 cookie: 1 fruit exchange 1 fat exchange		
	Protein	1 gm
	Fat	4 gm
	Carbohydrate	8 gm
	Sodium	52 mg
	Potassium	8 mg
	Calories	72

2 cookies: 1 bread-starch exchange 1½ fat exchanges		
	Protein	2 gm
	Fat	8 gm
	Carbohydrate	16 gm
	Sodium	104 mg
	Potassium	16 mg
	Calories	144

Marshmallow Dainties

3 squares bittersweet chocolate (3 oz)
2 eggs
1 cup powdered sugar
1 tsp vanilla
pinch of salt
1 cup chopped nuts
2½ cups miniature marshmallows
1 cup toasted coconut

1. Melt chocolate. Add beaten eggs.

2. Add remaining ingredients.

3. Drop by teaspoonfuls in dish of toasted coconut.

Yield: 40 cookies

1 cookie: ½ fruit exchange 1 fat exchange		
Protein	1 gm
Fat	4 gm
Carbohydrate	7 gm
Sodium	7 mg
Potassium	36 mg
Calories	68

2 cookies: 1 bread-starch exchange 1½ fat exchanges		
Protein	2 gm
Fat	8 gm
Carbohydrate	14 gm
Sodium	14 mg
Potassium	72 mg
Calories	136

Merry Christmas Cut-Out Cookies

1 cup butter or margarine
¾ cug granulated sugar
1 egg
1 tsp vanilla
2¾ cups sifted all-purpose flour
½ tsp salt
1 cup quick uncooked oats

1. Beat butter until creamy.

2. Gradually add sugar, beating until fluffy.

3. Add eggs.

4. Blend in vanilla.

5. Sift together flour and salt. Add to creamed mixture. Blend well.

6. Stir in oats.

7. Chill dough at least one hour before rolling out.

8. Roll out on lightly floured board or canvas to ⅛ inch thickness.

9. Cut into desired shapes with floured cookie cutter.

10. Place on greased cookie sheets.

11. Bake in a preheated moderate oven at 350 degrees about 10–12 minutes.

12. Cool.

13. Decorate with confectioner's sugar frosting.

Yield: 6 dozen (72) cookies

1 cookie: ½ fruit exchange
　　　　 ½ fat exchange

Protein	1 gm
Fat	3 gm
Carbohydrate	6 gm
Sodium	54 mg
Potassium	10 mg
Calories	55

2 cookies: 1 fruit exchange
　　　　　 1 fat exchange

Protein	1 gm
Fat	6 gm
Carbohydrate	12 gm
Sodium	108 mg
Potassium	20 mg
Calories	106

Cherry Delights

1 cup margarine
½ cup sugar
½ cup Karo Light Corn Syrup
2 egg yolks
2 egg whites
2½ cups flour
2 cups nuts, finely chopped
24 candied cherries, halved

1. Mix margarine and sugar.

2. Stir in Karo Syrup, egg yolks, and flour.

3. Chill.

4. Roll into 1 inch balls.

5. Mix egg whites and nuts.

6. Dip each ball into egg white mixture.

7. Press ½ cherry into each ball.

8. Bake on greased cookie sheet at 325 degrees for 20 minutes.

Yield: 4 dozen cookies

2 cookies:	1 bread-starch exchange	Protein	4 gm
	1 fruit exchange	Fat	10 gm
	2 fat exchanges	Carbohydrate	22 gm
		Sodium	96 mg
		Potassium	30 mg
		Calories	194
1 cookie:	1 fruit exchange	Protein	2 gm
	1 fat exchange	Fat	5 gm
		Carbohydrate	11 gm
		Sodium	48 mg
		Potassium	15 mg
		Calories	97

Date Cookies

1¼ cups water
2 cups dates, chopped
2 tsp cinnamon
⅓ cup shortening
½ tsp nutmeg
2 beaten eggs
1 tsp baking soda
½ tsp salt
2 tbsp water
1¼ tsp liquid sugar substitute
2 cups flour
1 tsp baking powder

1. Combine 1¼ cups of water with dates, cinnamon, shortening, and nutmeg.

2. Boil for 3 minutes and cool.

3. Add eggs, soda, salt, 2 tbsp water, and liquid sweetener. Stir well then add flour combined with baking powder.

4. Drop with a teaspoon onto a greased baking sheet. Bake 12–15 minutes at 350 degrees.

Yield: 3 dozen
1 cookie: 1 bread-starch exchange

Protein	1 gm
Fat	2 gm
Carbohydrate	13 gm
Sodium	63 mg
Potassium	75 mg
Calories	74

Chocolate Bon Bons

1 cup dates, finely chopped
1 cup chunky-style peanut butter
1 cup powdered sugar
1 cup nuts, chopped
1 tbsp butter

Topping

2 squares semi-sweet chocolate
1-6 oz package chocolate chips
1 inch square parafin

1. Mix together cookie ingredients.

2. Roll into small balls (1 inch in diameter).

3. Melt semi-sweet chocolate and chocolate chips in double boiler.

4. Melt parafin.

5. Add parafin to chocolate mixture.

6. Dip balls into chocolate mixture.

Yield: 60 cookies
2 cookies: 1 bread-starch exchange
            2 fat exchanges

Protein	3 gm
Fat	10 gm
Carbohydrate	14 gm
Sodium	56 mg
Potassium	136 mg
Calories	158

Pecan Brittle

1½ cups chopped pecans
2 cups sugar

1. Spread 1½ cups coarsely chopped pecans in a shallow baking pan. Toast in a 350 degree oven for 10 minutes.

2. Grease a 15½x10½ inch shallow pan or marble slab.

3. In a heavy skillet, heat 2 cups sugar over medium-low heat, stirring constantly with a wooden spoon, until sugar melts and has a golden color. About 18–20 minutes.

4. Stir in the pecans.

5. Immediately pour into a greased pan or onto a marble slab.

6. Quickly spread using a greased spatula.

7. Cool until solid.

8. Break into pieces.

Yield: 1½ pounds candy (24 ounces)
1 ounce (24 servings):

2 fruit exchanges	Protein	0 gm
1 fat exchange	Fat	5 gm
	Carbohydrate	18 gm
	Sodium	0 mg
	Potassium	45 mg
	Calories	117

½ ounce (48 servings):

1 fruit exchange	Protein	0 gm
½ fat exchange	Fat	2 gm
	Carbohydrate	9 gm
	Sodium	0 mg
	Potassium	22 mg
	Calories	54

Peanut Brittle

2 cups sugar
1 cup light corn syrup
1 cup water
2 cups raw Spanish peanuts
½ tsp salt
1 tbsp butter or margarine
1 tsp baking soda

1. In heavy 3 quart saucepan, combine sugar, light corn syrup, and water.

2. Cook and stir until sugar dissolves.

3. Cook over medium heat to a soft ball stage.

4. Stir in raw Spanish peanuts and salt.

5. Cook to hard crack stage (350 degrees), stirring frequently.

6. Stir in butter or margarine and baking soda. (Mixture will bubble.)

7. Pour at once into 2 well-buttered cookie sheets, spreading with a spatula.

8. If desired, cool slightly and pull with forks to make thinner.

9. Break into pieces when cool.

Yield: 1½ pounds of candy (24 ounces)
1 serving (24 servings):

1 bread-starch	Protein	3 gm
exchange	Fat	6 gm
1 fruit exchange	Carbohydrate	27 gm
1 fat exchange	Sodium	112 mg
	Potassium	82 mg
	Calories	174

½ serving (48 servings):

1 bread-starch	Protein	1 gm
exchange	Fat	3 gm
½ fat exchange	Carbohydrate	13 gm
	Sodium	56 mg
	Potassium	41 mg
	Calories	83

Caramel Corn

3¾ quarts (15 cups) popped corn (large kernel corn)
1 cup packed brown sugar
½ cup margarine
¼ cup light corn syrup
½ tsp salt
½ tsp soda

1. Preheat oven to 200 degrees.

2. Divide popped corn between 2 ungreased baking pans, 13 x 9 x 2 inches.

3. Heat sugar, margarine, corn syrup, and salt, stirring occasionally until bubbly around edges.

4. Continue cooking over medium heat for 5 minutes.

5. Remove from heat.

6. Stir in soda until foamy.

7. Pour on popped corn, stirring until corn is well coated.

8. Bake 1 hour, stirring every 15 minutes.

Yield: 15 cups

1 cup: 2 fruit exchanges	Protein	1 gm
1½ fat exchanges	Carbohydrate	22 gm
OR	Fat	8 gm
	Sodium	162 mg
1 bread-starch exchange	Potassium	52 mg
1 fruit exchange	Calories	164
1½ fat exchange		

Chow Mein Noodle Candy

½ cup chow mein noodles
3 large marshmallows
12 Virginia peanuts
4 tbsp low-calorie chocolate syrup

1. Melt marshmallows in the top of a double boiler.

2. Mix in noodles and peanuts.

3. Drop by spoonful onto waxed paper.

4. Drizzle low calorie chocolate syrup on top of each candy.

5. Chill.

Yield: 8 pieces of candy
2 pieces: 1 fat exchange
          1 fruit exchange

Protein	3 gm
Fat	5 gm
Carbohydrate	10 gm
Sodium	38 mg
Potassium	46 mg
Calories	97

Chocolate Caramels

2 cups sugar
1 cup butter
1 cup corn syrup
2 cups cream (half & half)
3 squares bittersweet chocolate (3 ounces)
1 cup walnuts, chopped

---

1. Mix sugar, butter, and corn syrup with 1 cup of cream in 4-quart kettle. Bring to a boil.

2. Then add second cup of cream. Cook to hard ball stage.

3. Remove from heat and add melted chocolate and nuts.

4. Pour in buttered pan, 10x2x15 inches.

5. Cut in one-inch squares.

Yield: 150 one-inch squares

1 square: ½ fruit exchange ½ fat exchange		
Protein	0 gm
Fat	3 gm
Carbohydrate	5 gm
Sodium	16 mg
Potassium	12 mg
Calories	47

2 squares: 1 fruit exchange 1 fat exchange		
Protein	0 gm
Fat	5 gm
Carbohydrate	10 gm
Sodium	32 mg
Potassium	24 mg
Calories	85

Fudge

4½ cups white sugar
1-14 oz can Carnation evaporated milk
4 packages (48 oz) chocolate chips
1-7 oz jar marshmallow creme
2 tsp vanilla
2 cups walnuts, chopped
¼ tsp salt
¼ cup butter or margarine

1. Put marshmallow and chips into large bowl.

2. Place sugar and milk in pan.

3. Cook to a rolling boil. Boil 4½ minutes.

4. Pour over chips and marshmallow.

5. Add salt and margarine. Stir until melted.

6. Add vanilla and nuts.

7. Put in a 13 x 9 inch pan and chill until firm.

8. Cut into 1 inch squares.

Yield: 107 pieces

1 piece:	1½ fruit exchanges	Protein	1 gm
	1 fat exchange	Fat	7 gm
	OR	Carbohydrate	17 gm
		Sodium	16 mg
	1 bread-starch exchange	Potassium	65 mg
	1 fat exchange	Calories	135

Molasses Taffy

2 tsp butter
2 cups sugar
1 cup light molasses
⅓ cup water
2 tsp vinegar
2 tbsp butter
½ tsp baking soda

1. Butter sides of heavy 3-quart saucepan.

2. In saucepan, mix sugar, molasses, and water.

3. Heat slowly, stirring constantly, until boiling.

4. Stir in vinegar, cook mixture to soft crack stage (270 degrees).

5. Remove from heat.

6. Add 2 tablespoons of butter.

7. Sift in soda and mix.

8. Pour into buttered 15½ x 10½ x 1 inch pan.

9. Cool until mixture is easy to handle.

10. Butter hands.

11. Gather taffy into a ball. Pull.

12. When golden and hard to pull, cut in fourths.

13. Pull into strands about ½ inch thick.

14. With buttered scissors, snip into bite-size pieces.

15. Wrap in wax paper.

Yield: 1¼ pounds (20 ounces)
1 ounce: 3 fruit exchanges

Protein	0 gm
Fat	1 gm
Carbohydrate	30 gm
Sodium	28 mg
Potassium	152 mg
Calories	129

½ ounce: 1½ fruit exchanges

Protein	0 gm
Fat	0 gm
Carbohydrate	15 gm
Sodium	14 mg
Potassium	76 mg
Calories	60

Divinity

3 egg whites (⅓ cup)
3 cups sugar
⅔ cup light corn syrup
¼ tsp salt
1 tsp vanilla extract
1 cup coarsely chopped pecans
6 candied cherries, quartered

1. Turn egg whites into large bowl of electric mixer. Let warm to room temperature for 1 hour.

2. Line an 11 x 7 x 1½ inch pan with waxed paper.

3. In heavy, 3-quart saucepan, combine sugar and corn syrup with ¾ cup water. Cook stirring over low heat to dissolve sugar. Cover. Cook 1 minute longer to dissolve sugar crystals on side of pan.

4. Uncover. Bring to a boil. Without stirring, cook to 260 on candy thermometer, or when a small amount of cold water forms a ball hard enough to hold its shape. Let cool slightly.

5. When candy thermometer goes down to 150 degrees beat egg whites with salt added until stiff peaks form when beater is slowly raised.

6. Gradually, pour hot syrup over egg whites in a thin stream beating constantly at a high speed until stiff peaks form when beater is raised—about 5 minutes.

7. Using a wooden spoon, beat in vanilla, chopped pecans, and quartered cherries. Continue beating until mixture is stiff enough to hold its shape and looks dull.

8. Turn into prepared pan. Do not scrape saucepan. Let stand until firm. With sharp knife, cut into 24 pieces. Store in wax paper. Keep in a closed container. Will keep for at least one week.

Yield: 24 pieces
1 piece: 3 fruit exchanges
      ½ fat exchange

Protein	1 gm
Fat	3 gm
Carbohydrate	32 gm
Sodium	29 mg
Potassium	37 mg
Calories	159

BEVERAGES

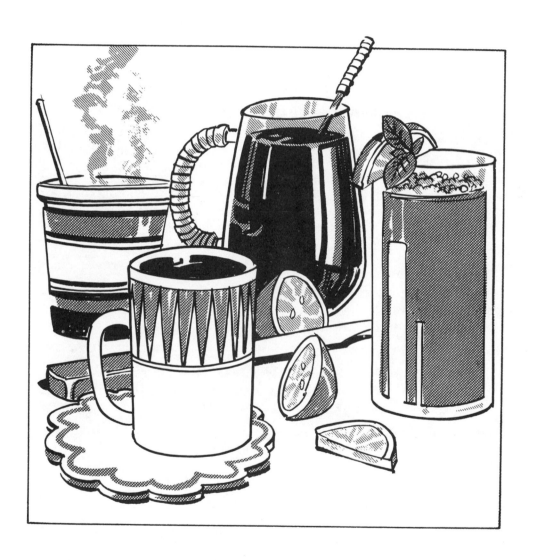

Lemonade

3 tbsp lemon juice
¾ cup water
⅜ tsp liquid artificial sweetener

1. Combine lemon juice, water, and liquid artificial sweetener.

2. Pour over crushed ice.

3. Garnish with lemon slice.

Yield: 1 serving
1 serving: free food exchange

Protein	0 gm
Fat	0 gm
Carbohydrate	4 gm
Sodium	0 mg
Potassium	63 mg
Calories	16

Limeade

½ cup unsweetened lime juice
1½ cups water
½ tbsp liquid artificial sweetener

1. Combine and add 1 pint sparkling water and green tinted ice cubes.

Yield: 4 servings (2 cups)
1 cup: free food exchange

Protein	0 gm
Fat	0 gm
Carbohydrate	5 gm
Sodium	0 mg
Potassium	64 mg
Calories	20

2 cups: 1 fruit exchange

Protein	0 gm
Fat	0 gm
Carbohydrate	11 gm
Sodium	0 mg
Potassium	128 mg
Calories	44

Tropical Sparkle

3 cups cold water
½ cup lime juice
½ cup lemon juice
2½–3 tsp liquid artificial sweetener
1 quart sugar free lemon-lime carbonated beverage
  chilled orange slices

1. Combine in punch bowl: water, lime juice, lemon juice, and liquid artificial sweetener.

2. Just before serving, add carbonated beverage and crushed ice.

3. Garnish with orange slices.

Yield: 2 quarts (8 cups)

1 cup: free food exchange		
Protein	0 gm
Fat	0 gm
Carbohydrate	2 gm
Sodium	28 mg
Potassium	37 mg
Calories	8

2 or 3 cups: ½ fruit exchange		
Protein	0 gm
Fat	0 gm
Carbohydrate	6 gm
Sodium	84 mg
Potassium	111 mg
Calories	24

4 cups: 1 fruit exchange		
Protein	0 gm
Fat	0 gm
Carbohydrate	8 gm
Sodium	112 mg
Potassium	148 mg
Calories	32

Cranberry Punch

2 cups low calorie cranberry juice
12 ounce can artificially sweetened lemon-lime flavored pop or
   soft drink
lemon slices

1. Combine cranberry juice and pop or soft drink.

2. Chill.

3. Serve in punch glasses.

4. Garnish with lemon slice.

Yield: 3½ cups

1 serving (7 ounces): ½ fruit exchange		
Protein	0 gm
Fat	0 gm
Carbohydrate	5 gm
Sodium	33 mg
Potassium	12 mg
Calories	20

Lemon Fizz

¾ cup sparkling water
3 tbsp lemon juice
⅜ tsp liquid artificial sweetener

1. Combine lemon juice, sparkling water, and liquid artificial
   sweetener.

2. Pour over crushed ice.

3. Garnish with lemon slice.

Yield: 1 serving

1 serving: free food exchange		
Protein	0 gm
Fat	0 gm
Carbohydrate	4 gm
Sodium	0 mg
Potassium	63 mg
Calories	16

Sparkling Cranberry Punch

2 cups ice water
½ cup lemon juice
2 cups low calorie lemon juice
1 tbsp liquid artificial sweetener
2 cups low calorie ginger ale, or club soda

1. Combine all ingredients.

2. Garnish with lemon or lime slices.

Yield: 6½ cups
1 cup: ½ fruit exchange

Protein	0 gm
Fat	0 gm
Carbohydrate	5 gm
Sodium	22 mg
Potassium	34 mg
Calories	20

Fruit Punch

¼ cup grape juice
¾ cup artificially sweetened lemon-lime flavored pop or soft
   drink

1. Mix all ingredients.

Yield: 2 servings (1 cup)
½ cup: ½ fruit exchange

Protein	0 gm
Fat	0 gm
Carbohydrate	5 gm
Sodium	21 mg
Potassium	37 mg
Calories	20

Ruby Slipper

3½ cups low calorie cranberry juice cocktail
1 cup unsweetened apple juice
¼ cup lemon juice
1¼ tsp liquid artificial sweetener
6 drops red food coloring
¼ tsp cinnamon
⅛ tsp salt
⅛ tsp cloves
⅛ tsp allspice

1. Combine all ingredients in 1½ quart sauce pan.

2. Heat to boiling.

3. Serve hot with cinnamon sticks if desired.

Variation for a clearer beverage:

1. Omit ground spices.

2. Add 2 cinnamon sticks and ½ tsp whole cloves.

3. Simmer 5 minutes.

4. Strain and serve.

Yield: 5 cups
1 serving (1 cup): 1½ fruit
   exchanges

Protein	0 gm
Fat	0 gm
Carbohydrate	15 gm
Sodium	70 mg
Potassium	84 mg
Calories	60

Hot Spiced Cider

2⅔ cups apple cider or apple juice
½ tsp allspice
6 whole cloves
1 (2 inch) cinnamon stick

1. Combine ingredients in saucepan.

2. Bring to a boil.

3. Strain into heated glass and serve.

Yield: 4 servings
1 serving—⅔ cup: 2 fruit exchanges

Protein	0 gm
Fat	0 gm
Carbohydrate	19 gm
Sodium	1 mg
Potassium	166 mg
Calories	76

Sparkling Strawberries

1 tsp liquid artificial sweetener
1 pint fresh strawberries, cut in half
1 cup chilled, sugar free lemon-lime carbonated beverage

1. Sprinkle liquid artificial sweetener over strawberries.

2. Pour carbonated beverage over strawberries just before serving.

Yield: 4 servings
1 serving: ½ fruit exchange

Protein	0 gm
Fat	0 gm
Carbohydrate	6 gm
Sodium	8 mg
Potassium	144 mg
Calories	24

Wassail

6 cups apple cider or juice
1 cinnamon stick or ¾ tsp cinnamon
¼ tsp nutmeg
¼ cup honey
3 tbsp lemon juice
1 tsp lemon peel, grated
2¼ cup unsweetened pineapple juice

1. Heat cider and cinnamon to boiling. Reduce heat. Cover and simmer 5 minutes.

2. Uncover and stir in remaining ingredients.

Yield: 6 cups

½ cup: 2½ fruit exchanges

Protein	0 gm
Fat	0 gm
Carbohydrate	27 gm
Sodium	2 mg
Potassium	204 mg
Calories	108

¼ cup: 1 fruit exchange

Protein	0 gm
Fat	0 gm
Carbohydrate	13 gm
Sodium	0 mg
Potassium	102 mg
Calories	52

Padré Punch

1-6 ounce can frozen orange juice, partially thawed
3 orange juice cans of water
1 quart apple cider or apple juice
5 whole cloves
2 cinnamon sticks
1 tsp ground nutmeg
¾ tsp ground ginger
orange slices

1. Combine all ingredients, except orange slices.

2. Heat to boiling. Reduce heat and simmer.

3. Garnish with orange slices.

Yield: 14-4 oz servings or 19-3 oz
          servings

4 oz serving: 1½ fruit exchanges

Protein	1 gm
Fat	0 gm
Carbohydrate	16 gm
Sodium	1 mg
Potassium	224 mg
Calories	68

3 oz serving: 1 fruit exchange

Protein	0 gm
Fat	0 gm
Carbohydrate	12 gm
Sodium	1 mg
Potassium	165 mg
Calories	48

Ginger Peachy Sodas

2 cups fresh or canned artificially sweetened peach slices,
    drained
1 pint vanilla ice milk
½ tsp ginger
½ tsp liquid artificial sweetener
1 quart bottle low-calorie ginger ale

1. Put peaches, ice milk, ginger and liquid artificial sweetener in blender.

2. Cover and blend on high speed for 30 seconds.

3. Fill four tall glasses half full. Add ginger ale.

Yield: 4 servings (4 cups)

1 serving: 1 bread-starch exchange		
1 bread-starch exchange	Protein	3 gm
	Fat	7 gm
1 fruit exchange	Carbohydrate	23 gm
1 fat exchange	Sodium	92 mg
	Potassium	287 mg
	Calories	167

Holiday Punch

1 package strawberry or cherry Kool-aid
liquid artificial sweetener to taste
2 cups club soda
2 cups low-calorie ginger ale
4 cups water

1. Combine all ingredients and garnish with orange slice.

Yield: 12 servings (6 cups)

½ cup-free food exchange		
½ cup-free food exchange	Protein	0 gm
	Fat	0 gm
	Carbohydrate	0 gm
	Sodium	0 mg
	Potassium	8 mg
	Calories	0

Christmas Egg Nog

1 egg
1 cup milk
¼ tsp vanilla
liquid artificial sweetener to taste
dash of nutmeg

1. Beat egg until thick and lemon colored.

2. Add milk, vanilla, and artificial sweetener.

3. Beat well.

4. Pour into a glass and sprinkle with nutmeg.

Yield: 1 serving
1 serving: 1 meat, medium-fat
   exchange
1 whole milk exchange

Protein	14 gm
Fat	16 gm
Carbohydrate	12 gm
Sodium	183 mg
Potassium	416 mg
Calories	248

New Year's Eggnog

⅓ cup sugar
2 egg yolks
4 cups milk, whole
2 egg whites
3 tbsp sugar
1 tsp vanilla
brandy or rum flavoring
ground nutmeg

1. Beat the ⅓ cup sugar into egg yolks. Add ¼ tsp salt. Stir into milk.

2. Cook and stir over medium heat until mixture coats a metal spoon. Cool.

3. Beat egg whites until foamy. Gradually add the 3 tbsp sugar, beating to soft peaks.

4. Add to egg mixture and mix well.

5. Add vanilla and flavoring to taste.

6. Chill.

7. Pour egg mixture into punch bowl. Sprinkle with nutmeg.

Yield: 8 (4 ounce) servings
½ cup: 2 fruit exchanges
      1 meat, low-fat
        exchange

OR

1 bread-starch exchange
½ fruit exchange
½ meat, medium-fat
   exchange
½ cup with 1 ounce
   brandy or rum: add 2 fat
   exchanges

Protein	5 gm
Fat	2 gm
Carbohydrate	19 gm
Sodium	142 mg
Potassium	192 mg
Calories	114

Orange Milk Shake

¼ cup milk, powdered, nonfat
½ cup orange juice

1. Place orange juice in a bowl.

2. Add ¼ cup of water if desired.

3. Place the milk powder in the orange juice.

4. Mix with a fork until there are no lumps.

5. Chill and serve at once.

Yield: 1 serving
1 serving: 1 fruit exchange
          1½ cup skim milk
            exchange

Protein	12 gm
Fat	0 gm
Carbohydrate	28 gm
Sodium	160 mg
Potassium	771 mg
Calories	160

NOTE: This recipe may be changed, and pineapple, apricot, or peach juice used in place of the orange juice.

Cocoa

3 tbsp cocoa
¾ tsp liquid artificial sweetener
¹⁄₁₆ tsp salt
½ cup water
3 cups skim milk
¼ tsp vanilla

1. Combine ingredients except skim milk and vanilla in sauce pan.

2. Cook over medium heat, stirring constantly until mixture comes to a rolling boil.

3. Add skim milk.

4. Heat to just boiling.

5. Stir in ¼ tsp vanilla.

Yield: 4 servings (4 cups)
1 serving (1 cup): 1 skim milk
   exchange

Protein	7 gm
Fat	1 gm
Carbohydrate	11 gm
Sodium	124 mg
Potassium	328 mg
Calories	81

IV

In Addition

A Look Into The Future

RESEARCH

Some exciting diabetes research has occurred in this decade. Pancreas transplants have been made. More success has been achieved in the transplant of "beta cells" (the cells which produce insulin). An "artificial pancreas" has been designed. This pancreas senses the blood sugar level by a computer implant and then releases an exact amount of insulin into the body. Research continues in the unfolding story of how viruses can induce diabetes. One day, scientists may be able to develop a vaccine to prevent insulin-dependent diabetes. These efforts may someday provide an answer to better care of diabetes. At the present, vaccines are not ready for human use.

BE INFORMED

Stay informed about diabetes. One of the best ways to do this is to join your local diabetes association. By joining, you will receive newsletters and a magazine called *Diabetes Forecast*. The American Diabetes Association magazine *Diabetes Forecast* is a good source of news, personal stories, and ideas. The *Diabetes Forecast* will also give you up-to-date facts and help. Most local associations also have regular meetings for diabetics. In these meetings you can learn of new developments in diabetes as well as share experiences and get support from each other.

You may want to help research efforts. This can be done through volunteer work. Each year bazaars, bike-a-thons, dinners, and concerts are sponsored by the local associations to raise money for research and patient services. Your interest and help is needed. The American Diabetes Association also sponsors camps for children with diabetes in most states.

Do not be afraid to ask for help. The American Diabetes Association has many people who understand your concerns. There are 10 million diabetics in the United States. It is simple to find other people to talk to about your disease when you join your local chapter or affiliate. See the listing under Community Resources. Listed here are the 67 affiliates of the American Diabetes Association located in every state. In addition, there are 600 local ADA chapters. Help yourself to help others.

A VOCABULARY LIST OF "$10 WORDS"

beta cells—the cells in the pancreas which make insulin.

bladder—a balloon-shaped organ in the lower abdomen which stores urine.

calorie—a unit of heat that measures the amount of energy in food. A calorie is the amount of heat needed to raise the temperature of one kilogram of water, one degree centigrade (C).

carbohydrate—a nutrient that provides the largest source of energy. The types of carbohydrate are sugars, starches, and fiber.

catheter—a long, fine tube inserted into the body to inject or drain fluids from the body.

cell—a small unit of living matter; the human body is made up of billions of cells.

cholesterol—a fatty-like substance that we can eat and that is made in the liver. The body needs cholesterol for metabolism and to make hormones. It can be retained in the blood system and is found in animal fat like meat, fish, chicken, and eggs.

chronic—lifelong, cannot be cured.

circulation—blood flow.

complications of diabetes—changes which occur in the body systems as a result of diabetes (circulation to heart, eyes, kidneys, feet, skin; nerve changes).

cortisone—a drug that may raise blood sugars.

diabetes mellitus—a life-long disease in which the body does not use food properly. The disease can affect many body systems.

diabetic acidosis—see ketoacidosis.

diabetic coma—another term for ketoacidosis; unconsciousness which may occur if ketoacidosis is not treated.

exchange—one serving of food from one food group. Other names are unit, substitute, serving, portion, or choice.

ECG (electrocardiogram)—a graphic record of the electrical activity of the heart muscle.

fat—a nutrient that stores energy; carries vitamins A, D, E, and K around in the body; and insulates and protects the body. Fat improves the taste and smell of food. Our bodies can make fat from the extra protein or carbohydrate that we eat.

Glucagon—a substance which must be injected into the body to raise the blood sugar level. Glucagon may be used to treat insulin reactions.

glucose—a form of sugar.

glutose—a sweet, gel-like substance in a squeeze bottle used to treat insulin reactions.

gram—a unit of weight in the metric system. A gram is ⅟₂₈ of an ounce, or 28 grams equal one ounce. Gram may be written as "g" or "gm."

hyperglycemia—high blood sugar.

hyperosmolar coma—unconsciousness which may occur if the blood sugar goes very high. Usually there are no ketones present in the urine or blood.

hypoglycemia—low blood sugar.

hypoglycemic pill—see "Oral hypoglycemic pill."

insulin—a chemical (hormone) made by the pancreas. Insulin opens the cell doors to allow blood sugar to enter the cell and be used for energy.

insulin reaction—low blood sugar; hypoglycemia; may occur in diabetics who take oral agents or insulin if the blood sugar goes too low.

ketoacidosis—a build-up of sugar and ketones in the body which occurs when there is not enough insulin. See Diabetic coma.

ketones—a poison made when the body cells burn fat for energy.

labile diabetes—unstable blood sugar results. (Wide ranges of blood sugar results.)

metabolism—all of the physical and chemical changes and activities that take place in the body. All the food substances that enter the body are used in the cells. Some of these activities are breathing and growing, and some are for repair and maintenance of the body.

mineral—a solid compound that is found in nature. Minerals are a part of all cells and help form bones and teeth. Minerals are needed in the glands, nerves, and for water balance. The most common minerals are calcium, iron, magnesium, sodium, potassium, phosphorus, and zinc.

normal blood sugar—70–110 milligrams of sugar per 100 milliliters of blood (mg %); a measurement of the amount of sugar in the blood stream.

nutrient—a substance that is found in food. Nutrients supply the body with the elements that are needed for growth, body repair, and the maintenance of all activities.

ophthalmologist—a medical doctor who specializes in the disease and treatment of the eyes.

oral hypoglycemic pill—a pill which lowers the blood sugar.

pancreas—an organ on the left side of the body behind the stomach which makes insulin and other substances the body needs to digest food.

polyunsaturated fat—a fat that can have extra hydrogen added to it. Most of the time it is a liquid and comes from a vegetable. Some examples are soybean oil, safflower oil, sunflower oil, and corn oil.

protein—a nutrient that provides energy, builds tissue, helps to regulate body functions and acts as a buffer in the body. The largest amount of protein is from animal and dairy sources. There are small amounts of protein in vegetables and starches.

renal threshold—the level of blood sugar at which the kidneys begin to spill sugar into the urine.

saturated fat—a fat that cannot have any hydrogen added to it. Most of the time this fat is a solid. Saturated fat is found in animal fat, bacon, butter, some margarines, and coconut oil.

second-voided specimen—a fresh urine sample obtained by emptying the bladder, then within 10–15 minutes urinating again and saving the sample.

starch—a complex form of carbohydrate. Starch is found in plants and is changed to sugar in the body.

stress test—a diagnostic method used to determine the body's response to physical exertion (stress). This involves taking physiological measurements (ECG, blood pressure, pulse, breathing, etc.) while exercising.

symptom—a signal of disease or condition in the body (for example, shaking is a symptom of an insulin reaction).

vitamin—a substance that is found in food in small amounts. Most vitamins cannot be made in the body. Vitamins are used in metabolism, hormone function, energy reactions, and to maintain health. Vitamins include A, D, E, and K; thiamine, riboflavin, folic acid, pantothenic acid, and ascorbic acid or vitamin C.

COMMUNITY RESOURCES

1. American Diabetes Association (ADA)
   Bimonthly magazine: *Diabetes Forecast*
   Charge: $15.00 annual dues (includes membership in local ADA affiliate and subscription to *Diabetes Forecast*)
   $9.00 for subscription only
   Address: American Diabetes Association
   2 Park Avenue
   New York, New York 10016

Local address: Ask your nurse or dietitian or physician
Local telephone: See your local telephone book

2. Health Education Specialists, Diabetes
Metropolitan Medical Center
Address: 900 South 8th Street
           Minneapolis, MN 55404
Telephone: (612) 347-4654 or 347-3977

3. Contact your local hospital regarding whether they have a diabetes education program or a diabetes educator (nurse or dietitian) available to give you assistance.

AFFILIATE ASSOCIATIONS
OF THE
AMERICAN DIABETES ASSOCIATION, INC.

ADA, ALABAMA AFFILIATE, INC.
904 Bob Wallace Avenue, SW, Suite 222
Huntsville, AL 35801
205-533-5775

ADA, ALASKA AFFILIATE, INC.
715 L Street, Suite 4
Anchorage, AK 99501
907-276-3607

ADA, ARIZONA AFFILIATE, INC.
555 West Catalina Drive, Suite 16
Phoenix, AZ 85013
602-274-3514

ADA, ARKANSAS AFFILIATE, INC.
5422 West Markham
Little Rock, AR 72205
501-666-9481

ADA, NORTHERN CALIFORNIA AFFILIATE, INC.
255 Hugo Street
San Francisco, CA 94122
415-681-8014

ADA, SOUTHERN CALIFORNIA AFFILIATE, INC.
3460 Wilshire Boulevard, Suite 900
Los Angeles, CA 90010
213-938-7271

ADA, COLORADO AFFILIATE, INC.
2450 South Downing Street
Denver, CO 80210
303-778-7556

ADA, CONNECTICUT AFFILIATE, INC.
17 Oakwood Avenue
West Hartford, CT 06119
203-236-1948

ADA, DELAWARE AFFILIATE, INC.
2713 Lancaster Avenue
Wilmington, DE 19806
302-656-0030

ADA, WASHINGTON DC AREA AFFILIATE, INC.
4405 East-West Highway, Suite 403
Bethesda, MD 20014
301-657-8303

ADA, FLORIDA AFFILIATE, INC.
3101 Maguire Boulevard, Suite 288
Orlando, FL 32803
305-894-6664

ADA, GEORGIA AFFILIATE, INC.
1447 Peachtree Street, NE, Suite 810
Atlanta, GA 30309
404-881-1963

ADA, HAWAII AFFILIATE, INC.
510 South Beretania Street, #101
Honolulu, HI 96813
808-521-5677

ADA, IDAHO AFFILIATE, INC.
1528 Vista
Boise, ID 83705
208-342-2774

ADA, DOWNSTATE ILLINOIS AFFILIATE, INC.
965 North Water Street
Decatur, IL 62523
217-422-8228

ADA, NORTHERN ILLINOIS AFFILIATE, INC.
6 North Michigan Avenue, Suite 1202
Chicago, IL 60602
312-346-1805

ADA, INDIANA AFFILIATE, INC.
222 South Downey, Suite 320
Indianapolis, IN 46219
317-353-9226

ADA, IOWA AFFILIATE, INC.
1118 First Avenue, NE
Cedar Rapids, IA 52402
319-366-6884

ADA, KANSAS AFFILIATE, INC.
2312 East Central
Wichita, KS 67214
316-265-6671

ADA, KENTUCKY AFFILIATE, INC.
682 Teton Trail
Frankfort, KY 40601
502-223-2971

ADA, LOUISIANA AFFILIATE, INC.
619 Jefferson Highway, Suite 2B
Baton Rouge, LA 70806
504-927-7732

ADA, MAINE AFFILIATE, INC.
16 Fahey Street
Belfast, ME 04915
207-338-4417

ADA, MARYLAND AFFILIATE, INC.
3701 Old Court Road, Suite 19
Baltimore, MD 21208
301-486-5515

ADA, MASSACHUSETTS AFFILIATE, INC.
377 Elliot Street
Newton Upper Falls, MA 02164
617-965-2323

ADA, MICHIGAN AFFILIATE, INC.
23100 Providence Drive, Suite 475
Southfield, MI 48075
313-552-0480

ADA, MINNESOTA AFFILIATE, INC.
5400 Glenwood Avenue North
Minneapolis, MN 55422
612-546-9619

ADA, MISSISSIPPI AFFILIATE, INC.
3000 Old Canton Road, Suite 475
Jackson, MS 39216
601-981-9511

ADA, GREATER ST. LOUIS AFFILIATE, INC.
1780 South Brentwood Boulevard
St. Louis, MO 63144
314-968-3196

ADA, HEART OF AMERICA AFFILIATE, INC.
616 East 63rd Street, Suite 203
Kansas City, MO 64110
816-361-3361

ADA, MISSOURI REGIONAL AFFILIATE, INC.
811 Cherry
Columbia, MO 65201
314-443-8611

ADA, MONTANA AFFILIATE, INC.
600 Central Plaza, Suite 8
Great Falls, MT 59403
406-761-0908

ADA, NEBRASKA AFFILIATE, INC.
7377 Pacific, Suite 216
Omaha, NE 68114
402-391-1251

ADA, NEVADA AFFILIATE, INC.
252 Convention Center Drive
Las Vegas, NV 89109
702-735-6339

ADA, NEW HAMPSHIRE AFFILIATE, INC.
194 North Main Street
Concord, NH 03301
603-228-1116

ADA, NEW JERSEY AFFILIATE, INC.
345 Union Street
Hackensack, NJ 07601
201-487-7228

ADA, NEW MEXICO AFFILIATE, INC.
525 San Pedro, NE, Suite 100
Albuquerque, NM 87108
505-266-5716

ADA, CENTRAL NEW YORK CHAPTER, INC.
1404 Genesee Street
Utica, NY 13502
315-735-0591

ADA, NEW YORK DIABETES AFFILIATE, INC.
55 West 39th Street
New York, NY 10018
212-944-7899

ADA, ROCHESTER REGIONAL AFFILIATE, INC.
797 Elmwood Avenue
Rochester, NY 14620
716-271-1260

ADA, UPSTATE NEW YORK CHAPTER, INC.
306 South Salina Street
Syracuse, NY 13202
315-475-1228

ADA, WESTERN NEW YORK AFFILIATE, INC.
107 Delaware Avenue, Suite 240
Buffalo, NY 14202
716-847-0220

ADA, NORTH CAROLINA AFFILIATE, INC.
100 Station Plaza, Suite 210
Rocky Mount, NC 27801
919-446-1108

ADA, NORTH DAKOTA AFFILIATE, INC.
101 North 3rd Street, Suite 502
Grand Forks, ND 58201
701-746-4427

ADA, AKRON AREA AFFILIATE, INC.
255 West Exchange Street
Akron, OH 44302
216-762-7487

ADA, CINCINNATI AFFILIATE, INC.
1216 East McMillan Street
Cincinnati, OH 45206
513-221-2111

ADA, DAYTON AREA AFFILIATE, INC.
184 Salem Avenue
Dayton, OH 45406
513-225-3002

ADA, GREATER OHIO AFFILIATE, INC.
P.O. Box 432
Lancaster, OH 43130
419-423-7608

ADA, EASTERN OKLAHOMA CHAPTER, INC.
6565 South Yale Avenue, Suite 613
Tulsa, OK 74177
918-492-4047

ADA, WESTERN OKLAHOMA CHAPTER, INC.
2801 NW Expressway, Suite 146
Oklahoma City, OK 73112
405-842-8839

ADA, OREGON AFFILIATE, INC.
3607 SW Corbett
Portland, OR 97201
503-228-0849

ADA, GREATER PHILADELPHIA AFFILIATE, INC.
21 South Fifth Street, Suite 570
Philadelphia, PA 19106
215-627-7718

ADA, WESTERN PENNSYLVANIA AFFILIATE, INC.
4617 Winthrop Street
Pittsburgh, PA 15213
412-682-3392

ADA, MID-PENNSYLVANIA AFFILIATE, INC.
430 East Broad Street
Bethlehem, PA 18018
215-867-6660

ADA, RHODE ISLAND AFFILIATE, INC.
4 Fallon Avenue
Providence, RI 02908
401-331-0099

ADA, SOUTH CAROLINA AFFILIATE, INC.
2838 Devine Street
Columbia, SC 29205
803-799-4246

ADA, SOUTH DAKOTA AFFILIATE, INC.
Route 1, Box 134
Baltic, SD 57003
605-529-5639

ADA, GREATER TENNESSEE AFFILIATE, INC.
1121 21st Avenue South, Room 226
Nashville, TN 37212
615-320-0493

ADA, MID-SOUTH AFFILIATE, INC.
969 Madison Avenue, Suite 900-A
Memphis, TN 38104
901-522-9539

ADA, TEXAS AFFILIATE, INC.
6201 Middle Fiskville Road
Austin, TX 78752
512-454-7614

ADA, UTAH AFFILIATE, INC.
1174 East 2700 South, #4
Salt Lake City, UT 84106
801-486-4980

ADA, VERMONT AFFILIATE, INC.
37 Elmwood Avenue
Burlington, VT 05401
802-862-3882

ADA, VIRGINIA AFFILIATE, INC.
404 8th Street NE
Charlottesville, VA 22901
804-293-4953

ADA, WASHINGTON AFFILIATE, INC.
3201 Fremont Avenue North
Seattle, WA 98103
206-632-4576

ADA, WEST VIRGINIA AFFILIATE, INC.
1036 Quarrier Street, Room 404
Charleston, WV 25301
304-346-6418

ADA, WISCONSIN AFFILIATE, INC.
6915 West Fond du Lac Avenue
Milwaukee, WI 53218
414-464-9395

ADA, WYOMING AFFILIATE, INC.
Box 1433
Laramie, WY 82070
307-638-3578

GENERAL INFORMATION

Diabetes Education Package (for the diabetes educator)
Metropolitan Medical Center
900 South Eighth St.
Minneapolis, MN 55404
Price: $15.00 plus postage and handling
The six forms in this package have been developed to help in new diabetes education programs, or to supplement existing programs. The forms are copyrighted but you can reproduce them if credit is given to Metropolitan Medical Center. The six forms are:

1. A questionnaire
2. A client-completed profile
3. A behavior assessment and expected outcome guide

The areas incorporated in the forms are basic and essential. The first two parts are to be completed by the client and/or significant others. The forms are in large print to aid in reading and filling them out. The reading level of the questionnaire ranges from 5.92 to 9.5. This is directly correlated with the questionnaire which begins with the simpler questions and ends with the more difficult ones. The profile is at the 5.76 grade reading level. This could easily be converted to other languages for non-English speaking clients.

QUESTIONNAIRE

The questionnaire has three objectives: 1) to assess the client's knowledge. It assists the educator and the client in concentrating on specific areas of learning. 2) It can be used as a pre-test and post-test, consequently measuring change that occurs as a result of teaching. 3) To stimulate the client and/or significant other to learn more about diabetes.

CLIENT-COMPLETED PROFILE

The profile form provides a baseline of the client's management of diabetes. It can also express the learning needs of the client.

BEHAVIOR ASSESSMENT AND EXPECTED OUTCOME GUIDELINE

The guide provides criteria for a multidisciplinary approach to teaching and demonstrating the teaching process. It can be used on an in or outpatient basis. The information obtained from the client-completed profile can be transcribed onto the current practices column. It provides a teaching flow sheet for improved documentation of teaching. It is concise, simple, and behaviorally oriented. The educator and/or client writes in the date and his/her initials when explanation/demonstration is given and/or received.

If further documentation is needed to describe a technique or procedure, an asterisk, date, and initials are placed in the appropriate section.

This indicates that the explanation can be found in the charting and/or care plan. Another facet of the guide is that it can be used as a contract; the client knows what objectives are expected of him/her and he/she can indicate his/her objectives. Any additional information acquired can be added on the back of the sheet.

The other forms included in this package are:

4. A class objectives in a study question format
5. A content of classes offered
6. An insulin injection ratio site chart

Diabetic nurse and dietitian specialists are available as consultants in establishing and developing diabetes education programs. Please call the Metropolitan Medical Center or write for more information.

Guide for Healthful Eating

Metropolitan Medical Center
900 South Eighth St.
Minneapolis, MN 55404
Price: $0.25 plus postage and handling
Also available in Spanish

This is a large print, simplified meal plan to be used with clients who are unable to use the ADA Exchange List. This brochure contains:

—three pages, each containing a meal plan displayed as a place setting
—a page of free foods
—a clock diagram which tells when to eat each meal. The portion size has been changed to ½ cup for the fruit and bread-starch exchanges. The total amount for the meat exchange at one meal is written in during the instruction.

Daily Diabetes Control Record

Metropolitan Medical Center
900 South Eighth St.
Minneapolis, MN 55404
Price: $0.40 per copy or 12 for $4.00 plus postage and handling

Twelve monthly charts for diabetics to use for recording urine tests, medication, and comments.

Diabetes: Healthy Living, Healthy Eating, Healthy Future (for the diabetes educator)

Plexus Communications Corporation
15760 Ventura Boulevard, Suite 532
Encino, CA 91436
For information on prices contact Plexus at (800) 423-3061 or (213) 995-1947

This series of tapes can enhance your diabetes education program by offering these benefits:

—save hours in instructional time

—provides current, consistent, and high-quality information
—the audiovisual format adds interest and promotes learning
—the programs can be used for individual or group instruction
—all tapes are in color

Each tape coincides with a chapter in the book *Diabetes: Recipes for Health* to provide continuity and reinforcement.

Diabetes in the Family
American Diabetes Association
2 Park Avenue
New York, NY 10016
Price; $12.95 for hard cover plus $2.00 for postage and handling
          $8.95 for paperback plus $1.25 for postage and handling

The American Diabetes Association's new (1982) comprehensive reference book on diabetes, addressed to both the newly diagnosed and those who have had diabetes for some time, and to their families. A valuable handbook of information on all aspects of diabetes, treatment, control, psychological impact, and research.

Family Cookbook
American Diabetes Association
2 Park Avenue
New York, NY 10016
Price: $12.95 plus $2.00 for postage and handling

The American Diabetes Association's cookbook that features more than 250 delicious, economical, kitchen-tested recipes that the whole family will savor. In addition to recipes, it is an encyclopedia of nutrition information.

The "Other" Diabetes
American Diabetes Association
2 Park Avenue
New York, NY 10016
Price: $1.00 per copy

This booklet features information on Type II diabetes and its treatment.

INDEX

A

Acetest, 9
  use of, 11, 12
Acidosis, diabetic, *see* Ketoacidosis
Actrapid, 30
Adult onset diabetes, 6
Aerobic activity, exercise for, 25
Age, hyperosmolar coma and, 54
Alcoholic beverages, 105
  food substitution and, 105
  guidelines for use, 105–106
  insulin reaction and, 49
American Diabetes Association
        (ADA), 379–380, 383–384
  affiliate associations, 384–387
Artificially sweetened, labeling of,
        92
Aspartame, 90
Asymptomatic diabetes, 6

B

Bean(s), 79
Bean exchange, nutritional contents,
        82
Beta cells, transplant of, 379
Beverages, restaurant dining and,
        104
  see also Alcoholic beverages
bG Chemstrip, 13
Bladder infection, signs of, 132
Blood sugar, 4
  levels
    control of, 18, 19, 43
    high
      hyperosmolar coma and, 154
      signs of, 54
      symptoms of, 53
    ketoacidosis and, 51, 52, 53
    low, *see* Insulin reaction
    lowering of, alcohol and, 105
    normal, 4, 13
    raising of, insulin reaction and,
        48
    rise in, 4, 6
      during pregnancy, 6, 7

symptoms of, 6
  self testing of, see Self blood
  sugar testing
  in urine, 8
  manufacture of, 18
  movement into cells, 5f
  spilling into urine, 13
Blood vessels, changes in, 131
Body, effects of diabetes on, 3
Body weight
  control of, 18
  ideal, 19–20
    reaching of, 20
  loss of, 6
  see also Obesity
Borderline diabetes, 6
Bread(s), 79
  restaurant dining and, 104
Bread-starch exchange, 70f–71, 113,
        120
  illness and, 110
  nutritional contents, 80–81
Bread-starch group, 61, 79
Breathing, shallow, 54
Brittle diabetes, 6
Buerger-Allen exercises, 134–137
Bulk, 98
  see also Dietary fiber

C

Calorie(s)
  defined, 20
  low, labeling of, 91–92
  production of, 20–21
  reduced, labeling of, 92
Calorie level, factors in, 20
Carbohydrate(s), 60
  content in food, reading of, 91
  in diet, 20–21
  high carbohydrate, high fiber ex-
        change list, 78–83
  illness and, 109, 110–111
Cardiovascular endurance, exercise
        for, 25
Causes of diabetes, 3
Cell(s)

RECODES

C